MARSHALL LAW

Raw Foods to Red Meats

Where raw foodists, vegans, vegetarians and carnivores all share a seat at the same table.

"Whoever controls the shopping and the cooking, controls the health of the entire family". If your family members are fat or sick, you may want to take a close and serious look at the person doing the shopping, and the person preparing the family meals.

DETOX DAVE MARSHALL

www.DETOXOASIS.net   www.DETOXOASIS.me   www.FITBODYRETREAT.com

Copyright © 2012 by David Allen Marshall

Book design and copyediting by Ann Elizabeth Loughlin

All Rights Reserved

No part of this book may be reproduced in any form or by any electronic or mechanical means including information storage and retrieval systems, without permission in writing from the author. The only exception is by a reviewer, who may quote sort excerpts in a review.

Send inquiries to: ictdave@aol.com

Printed in the United States of America

First Printing: December 2012

Published by Elk Ridge, LLC

ISBN-10: 1481137336

ISBN-13: 978-1481137331

Contents

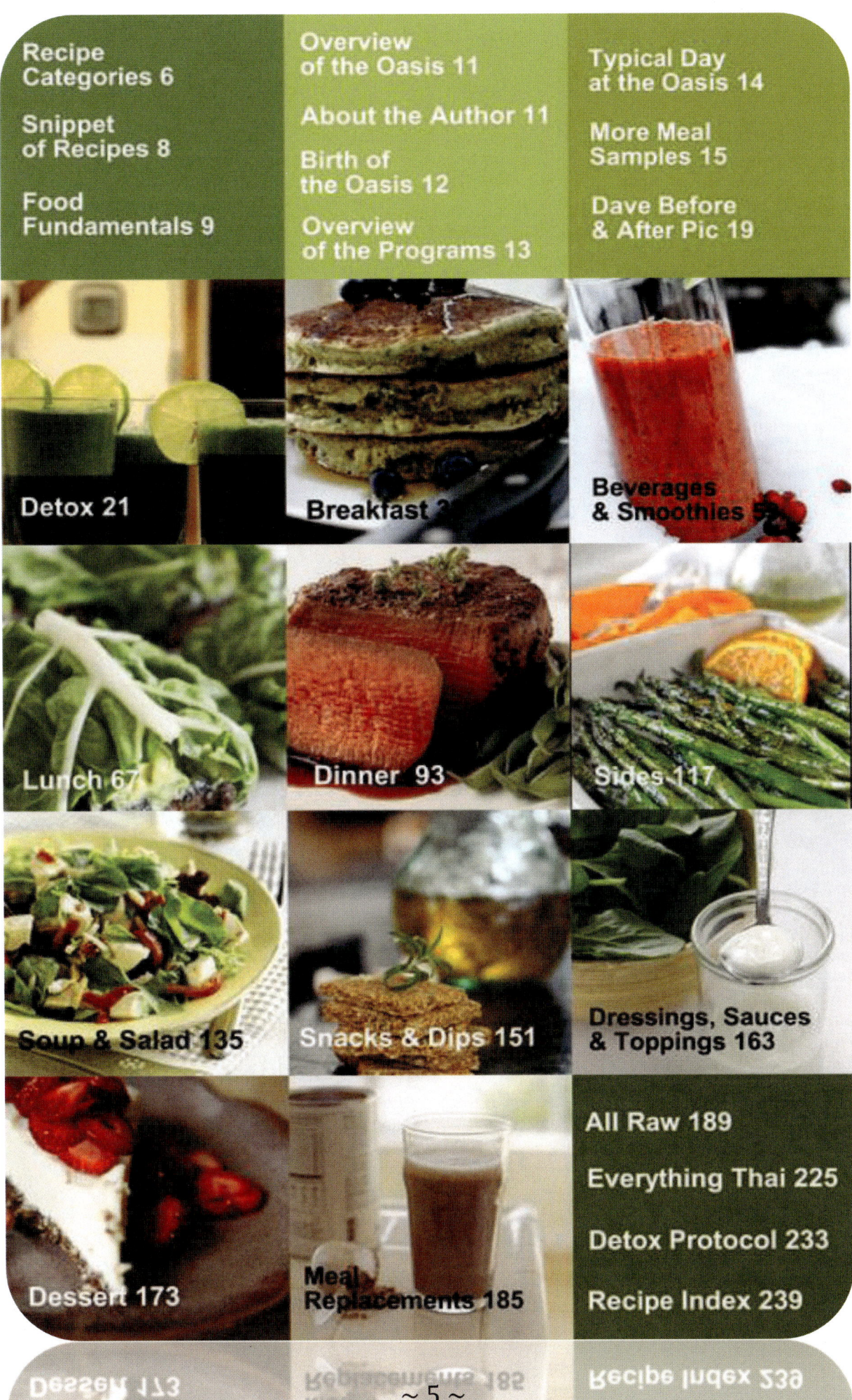

- Recipe Categories 6
- Snippet of Recipes 8
- Food Fundamentals 9
- Overview of the Oasis 11
- About the Author 11
- Birth of the Oasis 12
- Overview of the Programs 13
- Typical Day at the Oasis 14
- More Meal Samples 15
- Dave Before & After Pic 19
- Detox 21
- Breakfast
- Beverages & Smoothies
- Lunch 67
- Dinner 93
- Sides 117
- Soup & Salad 135
- Snacks & Dips 151
- Dressings, Sauces & Toppings 163
- Dessert 173
- Meal Replacements 185
- All Raw 189
- Everything Thai 225
- Detox Protocol 233
- Recipe Index 239

Recipe Categories

Detox

- Carrot, Apple & Green 22
- Greatest Detox Vegetable Broth 23
- Green Algae Drink 24
- Green Smoothie & Berries 25
- Green Veggie Juice #1 26
- Green Veggie Juice #2 27
- Growing Sprouts & Making Rejuvelac 28
- Liver Flush 29
- Psyllium & Bentonite Clay Drink 30
- Seaweed Mineral Drink 31

Breakfast

- Berries & Yogurt 34
- Breakfast Burritos 35
- Breakfast Quinoa 36
- Breakfast Tacos 37
- Cottage Cheese with Banana & Flax 38
- Eggs Easy & Quinoa 39
- Fage 2% Yogurt, Granola & Fresh Fruit 40
- Flaxseed Blueberry Pancakes 41
- French Toast 42
- Fresh Tomato Parmesan Scramble 43
- High Protein Oatmeal 44
- High Protein Pancakes 45
- Oaties & Scramble / Pico-de-Gallo 46
- Protein Omelet 47
- Scrambled Eggs with Cottage Cheese 48
- Scrambled Eggs with Feta & Veggie 49
- Scrambled Eggs with Goat Cheese & Red Peppers 50

Beverages & Smoothies

- Almond Nut Milk 54
- Carrot, Apple & Green 55
- Cocoa Almond Drink 56
- Green Algae Drink 57
- Green Smoothie & Berries 58
- Green Veggie Juice #1 59
- Green Veggie Juice #2 60
- High Power Smoothie 61
- Iced Herbal Coffee 62
- Real Orange & Fresh 63
- Seaweed Mineral Drink 64

Lunch

- Basil Grilled Chicken 68
- Beef Stew 69
- Buffalo Salsa Wrap 70
- Burrito Protein Power House 71
- Ceviche 72
- Chicken & Red Pepper Wrap 73
- Chicken Caesar Wrap 74
- Chicken Tofu Pizza 75
- Elk & Lentil Burritos 76
- Elk Chili 77
- Elk Garlic BBQ Burger 78
- Fish Cakes 79
- Lettuce Tofu Veggie Wraps 80
- Lettuce Veggie Wraps 81
- Quinoa, Beans & Elk 82
- Raw-Fajita Alternative 83
- Raw-Garden Burgers 84
- Raw-Zucchini Pasta 85
- Red Pepper Stuffed & Chicken Salad 86
- Turkey Sandwich 87
- Turkey Sandwich - Multigrain 88
- Turkey-Elk-Buffalo-Beef Burger Grilled 89
- White Chili - Turkey 90

Dinner

- Basil Grilled Chicken 94
- Beef Stew 95
- Chicken Satay 96
- Elk Meat Loaf 97
- Garlic Teriyaki Edamame & Chicken 98
- Ginger Salmon with Wild Rice 99
- Grilled Wasabi Salmon 100
- Lemon Herb Chicken 101
- Mediciettes, Steak Appetizer with Bearnaise Sauce 102
- Perfect Filet Mignon 103
- Pork Tenderloin 104
- Prime Rib Tenderloin 105
- Quinoa Curry & Chicken 106
- Raw-Zucchini Pasta 107
- Salmon & Cucumber Quinoa Salad 108
- Seared Ahi Tuna 109
- Shrimp & Rice Penne Pasta 110
- Spaghetti Squash with Chicken Breast 111
- Thai-Garlic Chicken 112
- Thai-Spicy Easy Fish 113
- Turkey & Fruit 114
- Wasabi Salmon 115

Sides (grains)

- Brown Rice 120
- Forbidden Black Wild Rice 122
- Himalayan Red Rice 124
- Quinoa Basic 127
- Quinoa Curry 128
- Rice Pasta - Gluten Free, Wheat Free 130

Sides (legumes)

- Black Beans Basic 119
- Green Beans 123
- Lentils Basic 125
- Lentils with Tomatoes 126

Sides (vegetables)

Asparagus	118
Coconut Sweet Potato or Yam	121
Red Skin Potatoes Roasted	129
Snow Peas	131
Spinach, Wilted with Mushrooms	132
Steamed Broccoli	133

Soup & Salad

Bean Salad	136
Curry Split Pea Soup	137
Energy Soup	138
Ginger Cucumber Salad	139
Ginger Salmon Salad	140
Lentil Soup	141
Quinoa and Edamame Salad	142
Salmon & Cucumber Quinoa Salad	143
Spicy Black Bean Soup	144
Spinach Salad	145
Spinach, Cabbage & Tuna Salad	146
Spinach, Pepper & Cheese Salad	147
Thai-Green Curry Soup	148
Thai-Herb Salad	149

Snacks & Dips

Basil Pesto	152
Hard Boiled Eggs & Hummus	153
High Protein Chips & Salsa	154
Mexican Flax Crackers	155
Pico-de-Gallo	156
Protein Bars	157
Raw-Smokey Jalapeno Cheese Alternative	158
Raw-Taco's Tasty Meat Alternative	159
Veggies & Hummus Dip	160

Dressings, Sauces & Toppings

Bearnaise Sauce II	164
Dave's Favorite Raw Dressing	165
Pico-de-Gallo	166
Raw-Alfredo Sauce	167
Raw-Ranch Dressing	168
Raw-Sour Cream	169
Spaghetti Sauce	170
Zero Calorie Dressing	171

Dessert

Berries & Yogurt	174
Cinnamon Apple & Almond Ricotta	175
Coconut Rice & Mango	176
Fresh Mango Yogurt	177
Raw-Apple Sauce	178
Raw-Berry Cheesecake	179
Raw-Chocolate Avocado Mousse	180
Raw-Ice Cream Sundae	181
Raw-Oatmeal Cookies	182
Spicy Fruity Thai Sensation	183

Meal Replacements

Super Post Workout Shake	186
Peanut Butter Chocolate Banana Oatmeal Post Workout Shake	186
A Bit of Green	187
Typical Replacement Shake	187

All Raw

Almond Nut Milk	190
Basil Pesto	191
Bean Salad	192
Carrot, Apple & Green	193
Cocoa Almond Drink	194
Dave's Favorite Raw Dressing	195
Energy Soup	196
Ginger Cucumber Salad	197
Green Algae Drink	198
Green Smoothie & Berries	199
Green Veggie Juice #1	200
Green Veggie Juice #2	201
Lettuce Veggie Wraps	202
Mexican Flax Crackers	203
Pico-de-Gallo	204
Raw-Alfredo Sauce	205
Raw-Apple Sauce	206
Raw-Berry Cheesecake	207
Raw-Chocolate Avocado Mousse	208
Raw-Fajita Alternative	209
Raw-Garden Burgers	210
Raw-Ice Cream Sundae	211
Raw-Oatmeal Cookies	212
Raw-Ranch Dressing	213
Raw-Smokey Jalapeno Cheese Alternative	214
Raw-Sour Cream	215
Raw-Taco's Tasty Meat Alternative	216
Raw-Zucchini Pasta	217
Real Orange & Fresh	218
Seaweed Mineral Drink	219
Spicy Fruity Thai Sensation	220
Veggies & Hummus Dip	221
Zero Calorie Dressing	222

Everything Thai

Chicken Satay	226
Spicy Fruity Thai Sensation	227
Thai-Garlic Chicken	228
Thai-Green Curry Soup	229
Thai-Herb Salad	230
Thai-Spicy Easy Fish	231

HERE IS A SNIPPET OF THE 100 PLUS FITNESS AND DETOX RECIPIES IN THIS BOOK AND MEALS SERVED AT THE OASIS!

BREAKFAST

STEEL CUT OATMEAL
Steel cut oatmeal served with a scoop of protein powder (strawberry, chocolate, or vanilla); topped with berries and crushed walnuts; then sprinkled with cinnamon

OMELET / EGG BEATER OR 5:1 EGGS
Eggbeater or 5:1 ratio egg omelet- real cheese, slices of turkey breast and spinach; then topped with salsa

LUNCH

CHICKEN WRAPS
Two spinach tortilla wraps with chicken breast, real cheese, spinach, romaine, avocado and tomato; served with a side of salsa

SALMON LUNCH
Atlantic salmon, seasoned and baked; then served on a bed of quinoa with a side of broccoli

DINNER

MANGO & PEAR CHICKEN
Chicken breast simmered in a special recipe chipotle sauce; served on a bed of spinach; then topped with mangos and pears

REAL BEEF-MIDWEST BEST (raised on-site and grass-fed)
Prime cut beef tenderloin topped with mushrooms; then served with steamed carrots, snow peas and zucchini

SNACKS

GARLIC EDAMAME
Just like at the sushi bar, except we boil our soy beans in garlic powder, not salt

GRANOLA YOGART WITH BERRIES
Fat free vanilla yogurt topped with fresh berries; then sprinkled with granola

PLUS... HEAPS OF RAW FOODS AND DETOX RECIPIES!

"Food is either fun or fuel. If every meal you eat has to be a carb amusement park in your mouth, then you my friend are doomed to a life of large. Bread and beer are off the menu - at least until you reach goal!"

Food Fundamentals from Fit Body Retreat and Detox Oasis

The **Marshall Law Fit Foods** cookbook provides the food fundamentals to help you lose weight, reduce body fat, and maintain your newfound look. In this book, you will find the foods you need to eat to help build or maintain the lean, toned, sexy shape that you desire.

The **Marshall Laws** of food preparation and presentation are outlined in a simple to understand format in the following pages. Our fitness foods program comes from years of daily use at our Fit Body Retreat and Detox Oasis center. This book is not intended for beginners. This book was written for fitness experts and clients who have attended one of our retreats in the past. A solid understanding of calorie burn rates; daily amounts of protein, carbohydrates and fats; and exercise programs are required to make this book work for you.

The program at our main Indiana location is a small family business, managed by experts that produce results. If you are overweight, you can expect to lose up to 40 pounds in 30 days through structured fitness and eating programs at our center. If you are already lean and fit, you can expect to take your fitness and foods knowledge to the next level.

Our rapid detox and cleanse programs helps clients lose 12 to 22 pounds in just 6 short days. This method of fasting is excellent to renew both body and mind through our 6 to 10 day herbal detox programs.

The focus of the Fit Body Retreat at the Oasis is not only to educate clients on what to eat but also to incorporate hands-on instruction in the kitchen, and how to make food preparation an enjoyable daily experience. This is a hands-on real life, real learning experience.

As part of the food prep program, clients learn the **Marshall Laws** of long-term weight management and muscle building success by gaining hands-on cooking experience each and every day of their stay. This hands-on approach provides our clients with the confidence they need to return home and implement the dietary changes they need for themselves and their families.

At the Fit Body Retreat and Oasis centers, clients get 4 to 5 hours of daily fitness in addition to hands-on food and meal training. The fitness and food education gives our clients the most important **Marshall Law** of all - **KNOWLEDGE**.

To get the full **Marshall Law** experience, you may just need to attend one of our retreats. Try a few of the recipes for yourself. We hope to see you at one of our retreat centers soon!

"If you go to your heart for advice it will not lie to you!"

Right or Wrong? It is impossible to reach a fitness or weight loss goal eating garbage. You can lie to yourself if you must, but if you are an adult, please don't tell me or others that you don't know what's right from wrong regarding your food choices. Most of us know in our heart of hearts that when we put something in our mouth to eat, it's either going to help us reach our weight and fitness goals, or it will not. You make a conscious decision every time your hand goes to your mouth. If you know it's bad for your weight or fitness goal, then just don't eat it! There is a reason you feel guilty after eating garbage foods. You only let yourself down when you eat junk foods like Twinkies or french fries. Be strong when tempted with poor food choices. More importantly.... be smart about your food!

Living under **Marshall Law** requires some common sense! If you don't know the calories of what you choose to put in your mouth, then simply don't eat it. At the very least, don't eat it until you know the calories, protein, carbs and fats in that item.

Make this your personal rule: know the numbers in the foods before you consume them. Reaching any fitness and weight loss goal means managing protein, carbs, fats, calorie consumption and your daily burn rates.

Would you buy a house not knowing the interest rate? Of course not! So apply this rule to your foods. Know the numbers before you consume.

By now, most of us would agree that food is 80% of our fitness and weight loss success, and our gym time is a mere 20% of our success. Listen to your inner voice and use common sense when eating. And do what your heart tells you!

Marshall Law also applies when you absolutely, positively need to lose 15 pounds this week. Just come to the Oasis. In 6 short days we will send you home looking brand new!

The day is coming when <u>all</u> American corporations will wake up and make an attempt to help its employees with their fitness and health through education programs. When they make an investment in company paid health coaches and teach their employees how to eat, they will increase productivity and reduce their health care costs. The corporation of the future will offer bonuses, incentives and rewards for employees that take their health and fitness seriously.

Detox Dave - Marshall Law

"While fasting at Detox Oasis, you can expect your body to start healing itself in just a few days, rather than months or weeks required at other centers."

Overview of the Oasis

Detox Oasis is located in the heart of the Midwest, on the outskirts of French lick, Indiana. The Oasis sits on 120 acres. We have a large garden where we raise hops, wheat grass, sprouts and have one of the largest vineyards in the state of Indiana. We also raise elk for our grass fed red meat consumption

The Oasis is a retreat center that allows the client a variety of programs that promote better health. From a detox week to fitness foods classes and exercise, the Oasis is a tool many people use to achieve better health and fitness.

At the Oasis, you will find a large group of interesting people with a variety of backgrounds and beliefs on what foods are best to consume. It may be the only place of its type where raw foodists, vegans, vegetarians, carnivores and those who fast, all share the same table. And that's ok. At the Oasis, different beliefs are accepted on personal health and fitness. We all strive for the same goal -- "better health". Some of us just choose a different path to achieve this goal.

Another difference in the Oasis center is our fitness program. We guide our guests through several hours a day of intense weight lifting, yoga, hikes and cardio. At other centers, you often get just a light stretch or a yoga class. The Oasis offers our clients the opportunity to cleanse their body through detox and clean foods plus tone up like never before.

About the Author, Owner and Founder

Owner and founder, Dave Marshall, has been involved in fasting, cleansing, raw foods, wheatgrass and fitness since the mid 70's. His first trainer job was in 1981 in Portland, Oregon.

Beginning in his 30's, Dave traveled the world, staying at a variety of health retreats and centers. In the early days of his fitness quest he attended many, "*just eat healthy, just do yoga, just eat raw or vegan, and we may just lose five pounds this week*" retreats. At the Oasis, we average 16 pounds in six days for weight loss.

While boxing in Thailand with his oldest son Dan, he discovered that the fasting retreats in SE Asia created "miracles" in healing and weight loss much quicker than the raw foods centers that he attended in the USA. He was disillusioned that both the fasting centers of Asia and the raw foods centers in the USA refused to allow or even consider a blend of services and methodology with their programs. The owners of these centers seemed to treat their programs and methods more as a religion instead of the simple tools to improved health that they really are. Each center claimed their method was the only true path to better health and wellness.

The Birth of the Oasis

At the Detox Oasis and Fit Body Retreat, we have a very open-minded approach to fitness and weight loss. We believe there are many paths to reaching fitness, weight loss and improved health. At the Oasis, we blended the best methods and practices of the raw food retreats in the USA and those methods used in the fasting centers of SE ASIA. Then we polished off our program with an aftercare foods and diet program that is very much like Bill Phillips' Body-For-Life teachings. This program is for people like you and I that seek a no-nonsense maintenance program requiring little thought and that's highly effective.

The Detox Oasis is not a rehab center as most westerners might think of the term "detox center". A good herbal detox can cleanse your body from chemicals in foods, stress hormones, sugar and caffeine. Some clients find they can get their head clear in one short week and conquer their cravings of garbage foods, sugar, caffeine, colas, and carbs. After a good detox, most people find they can make better decisions regarding the next path they need to take to achieve long-term success.

At the Oasis center, we help people cleanse their bodies, lose weight and start a fitness program that they can take home with them, move forward with, and maintain. The key to a rapid fitness or weight loss jump-start program is to first detox and cleanse the body to prepare it for change. This is much like a re-boot on a computer. Most of us know that our typical western diet is loaded with too many carbohydrates and not enough nutrient rich foods.

At the Oasis, clients expect some weight loss with a good detox, and that's exactly what they get! The average weight loss is about 2 pounds a day. At the end of a 5 or 6 day program, you will look and feel better than you have in years! Many people lose 12-22 pounds in a 6 day cleanse.

Our rejuvenation specialists have years of experience. Some would say they work miracles. We hope to see you at the Oasis soon!

Detox Dave - Marshall Law

"Do not ask yourself what the world needs; ask yourself instead what makes you come alive. And then go and do that. Because what the world needs is people who have come alive." ~ Harold Whitman

A Short Overview of the Programs at the Oasis

1. Detox and Cleanse Program - 6 to 10 days (our most popular program is the 10 day detox)

2. Raw Foods Prep Program - 2 day structured classes (generally follows the detox program as a transition into raw foods)

3. Fit Foods Program - includes grass-fed meats and fish - 6 to 90 days (weight loss program)

4. Fit Foods Program - no meat; vegan or vegetarian options - 6 to 90 days (weight loss program)

5. Fit Foods Medically Supervised Hormone Evaluation and Replacement Program (based on the doctor's recommendations and your comfort level)

6. Yoga Only Retreats- spend a week doing yoga, meditation and eating vegan or vegetarian dishes

Our programs are varied to suit the needs and comfort levels of our clients. There are many ways to achieve weight loss, fitness and better health. Not everyone wants to be a raw foodist, a vegan or a vegetarian. Our approach to helping our clients achieve their goals is to introduce them to options that will help lead them to success.

This cookbook is just another tool in achieving success in fitness and health. It has been described by some of our competitive clients as their "unfair advantage" over the competition. We hope that you too will use this book as a tool to help you reach your fitness goals.

What if every item that you bought at the grocery store, liquor store, drive-thru, and restaurant was public record? What if your pharmacy prescriptions and the time you spent in the gym was made public as well? If this information were made public, would it help you put more effort into improving your foods and fitness?

Pretend for just 1 week that every item you purchase or that someone purchases for you to consume is public record. This includes all food, drink and drugs. It would be posted online with a detailed personal report of your consumption habits and then distributed via e mail to everyone you know.

A damn scary thought for most of us! I ask that you play this troubling game for 1 short week.

How to play: simply write down every item that goes into your mouth for just 1 short week. Review it and share it with your trainer. Make changes as necessary.

"What if your monthly health insurance premium was based on your weight, your body fat percentage, and the food items that you bought at the grocery store? Would you change your eating habits? Currently I pay about $500.00 a month for my health insurance through my employer. What if it was only $50.00 a month for health insurance if you were lean and fit? Would that motivate you? It would me! I predict that health insurance premiums will continue to rise at the same rate as the rise in weight of the general population."

A Typical Day at the Oasis

This will give you an idea of what to expect should you attend an Oasis retreat. It's also why we can claim weight loss numbers up to 22 pounds in a week and 40 pounds in just 30 days.

All of our programs follow the same general daily schedule. Most people participate in the hikes, yoga and exercise classes. These classes are not mandatory, but neither is losing weight or getting fit!

Those who participate in the entire program tend to get more out of the program than those that do not.

Remember -- like anything in this life, the same holds true with the Oasis retreats. The more you put into the program, the more you will get out of it.

	Detox Program	**Fit Body Program**
07:00am	Wheat grass or Algae drink	Wheat grass or Algae drink
07:30am	7k hike	7k hike
08:30am	Green juice – spinach/sprouts/celery	Protein shake
09:00am	Abs class	Abs class
09:30am	Group weight training	Group weight training
10:30am	30 minutes of cardio	30 minutes of cardio
11:30am	Green juice – spinach/sprouts/celery	Protein shake
12:00pm	Colonic	Optional colonic
01:00-3:00pm	REST TIME	REST TIME
03:00pm	Green juice – spinach/sprouts/celery	Protein shake
03:30pm	Yoga	Yoga
04:30-6:00pm	REST TIME	Hands-on in kitchen, assisting in meal prep
06:00pm	Dinner – clear veggie broth	Dinner – salmon, asparagus, quinoa
07:00pm	Wheat grass or Algae drink	30 minutes of cardio

Evening talks: Learn to sprout from seeds; discussions on fitness and foods, and exercise management with a busy lifestyle.

Activities: Golf, sauna, skin brushing, Aqua Chi, Massages, Reiki, gardening, hiking, swimming, canoeing nearby, historic tours at the French Lick Springs Resort.

The Primary Differences in the Programs at the Oasis

The big differences in our programs are the foods, the calories and eating program. The daily schedule and the fitness schedule is essentially the same. The basic question when you come to the Oasis is this: are you going to eat or fast?

- The detox client is consuming juices and herbs throughout the day
- The fitness foods client is eating four to six meals a day and/or doing protein shakes

"Are you digging your own grave with your teeth? When you look into your shopping cart at the grocery store, are you happy with the items you placed in your cart, or do you feel some guilt? Are you helping yourself and your family build healthy bodies, or are you helping them dig their own grave with their teeth? Stop the madness and end the cycle. You and your family can be lean and fit. It's up to you to make the positive change."

FIT BODY RETREAT MORNING FUEL SELECTIONS
(Just a few samples out of over 100 recipes here)

BREAKFAST

STEEL CUT OATMEAL
Steel cut oatmeal served with a scoop of protein powder (strawberry, chocolate, or vanilla); topped with berries, crushed walnuts; then sprinkled with cinnamon

OMELET/EGG BEATER OR 5:1 EGGS
Eggbeater or 5:1 ratio egg omelet- real cheese, slices of turkey breast and spinach; then topped with salsa

HONG KONG SPECIAL SCRAMBLED EGGS & COTTAGE CHEESE
5:1 ratio eggs scrambled sprinkled with chives, tomato; then topped with low fat cottage cheese (*taught to Dave by a client in Hong Kong*)

MAYAN SUPER CHARGER- STEAK & QUINOA
5:1-ratio eggs; placed upon on a scoop of Quinoa; then served with slices of lean beef fillet

PROTEIN QUICKIE
A Myoplex shake with ¼ cup strawberries or blue berries; blended and served

EGGS & CHICKEN WITH RICE
5:1 ratio eggs and chicken breast; served with brown rice and red peppers; then sprinkled with real cheese

BREAKFAST TACOS
Three corn tortillas with ground turkey, 5:1 ratio eggs, real cheese, spices, green onions and a splash of salsa

MEXICAN POWERHOUSE-BEANS & EGGS
5:1 eggs, two corn tortillas and a scoop of black beans and onion; then topped with real cheese.

FIT BODY RETREAT HEALTHY MID DAY FUEL SELECTIONS

These are all higher carb meals (your best choice to consume during the day)

LUNCHES

CHICKEN WRAPS
Two spinach tortilla wraps with chicken breast, real cheese, spinach, romaine, avocado and tomato; then served with a side of salsa

SALMON LUNCH
Atlantic salmon, seasoned and baked; then served on a bed of quinoa with a side of broccoli

BASIL LEMON TURKEY BREAST
Slices of turkey breast seasoned with lemon and basil; then served on a bed of brown rice and topped with asparagus

BUFFALO PASTA
A yummy red sauce with lean high protein farm raised ground bison; spiced with high antioxidant spices; then served on top of wheat and gluten free brown rice spaghetti

TURKEY LOAF
Turkey meat loaf; served with sweet potato; then topped with cinnamon with a side of broccoli

SPICY TILAPIA
Tilapia grilled with southwest spices; served up on a bed of quinoa with a side of snow peas and spaghetti squash

ELK PROTEIN OVERLOAD
Super lean high protein farm raised Elk steak, black beans, quinoa, real cheese and a variety of spices

FIT BODY RETREAT YUMMY DINNER FUEL SELECTIONS

These are all low-carb meals (your best choice to consume in the evening)

DINNERS

ELK RANCH CHILI
Super lean high protein farm raised elk, with tomatoes, black beans, celery and bell peppers with heaps of delicious southwest spices

THAI SALAD
Cabbage, red and yellow peppers, tomato, cucumber, green onion, lemon grass, carrots, a hint of jalapeño pepper, mixed together with Dave's special Thai dressing; then topped with Atlantic salmon fillet

COSTA RICA CEVICHE
Shrimp and tilapia marinated in lime juice mixed with red peppers, onion, cucumber, cilantro, and tomato; then served on a bed of spinach

MANGO & PEAR CHICKEN
Chicken breast simmered in a special recipe chipotle sauce; served on a bed of spinach; then topped with mangos and pears

REAL BEEF-MIDWEST BEST (raised on-site and grass-fed)
Prime cut beef tenderloin; topped with mushrooms; then served with steamed carrots, snow peas and zucchini

CHICKEN SATAY
Thin slices of chicken breast; sautéed with yellow curry, red and yellow peppers and a touch of garlic; then served with a side of crisp fresh spinach

ELK FAJITAS
Super lean high protein farm raised elk with caramelized bell peppers, onions, broccoli, carrots; then served on low-carb tortillas

CHICKEN SALAD
A bowl of spinach, cucumber, tomato, chicken breast; then served with a low fat dressing, or the Oasis Zero Calorie Dressing

***IT IS A DOCUMENTED FACT:** "80% of a person's fit, lean, trim body results are achieved through diet and some 20% of their results are derived through hard training and fitness. This said, the person that combines fitness with perfect foods will look and feel better than those with no fitness or exercise."*

FIT BODY RETREAT HEALTHY SNACKS - FUEL!

SNACKS

BLACK BEANS
Mildly seasoned with onions and a southwestern spice; mixed with wild rice to make a complete protein dish; then topped with cilantro and salsa

ELK TACOS
Three small corn tortillas with ground elk, real cheese, cilantro and salsa

GARLIC EDAMAME
Just like at the sushi bar, except we boil our soy beans in garlic powder, not salt

GRANOLA YOGART WITH BERRIES
Fat free vanilla yogurt topped with fresh berries; then sprinkled with granola

JUST MEAT
Your choice of 4- 6 oz. chicken breast, an elk burger, salmon fillet, turkey burger, or steak, etc.. (burger without the bun of course!)

FARM RAISED AND LOCAL FOODS: I prefer to use bison, elk and grass fed beef, line-caught fresh Alaskan salmon, and other healthy meats at my center. I try to shop as organic as possible from local growers at farmers markets. However, I am not a purest. When necessary, I'll go to any store and purchase a lesser quality of these meats rather than go without!

Example on this statement: Although I desire line-caught fresh Alaskan salmon for dinner tonight, due to my poor planning on this meal, I end up with a frozen salmon fillet from Wal-Mart. Regardless, I'm still having salmon for dinner! My point is this - don't go crazy trying to eat perfect foods. Strive to do the best you can. Strive to do better each week.

Don't get stressed out when your foods, workouts or schedule is not perfect. Just work with what you have on hand and try to do better daily. If you wait for things to be perfect before you make change, you may wait forever. Start today and improve as you go!

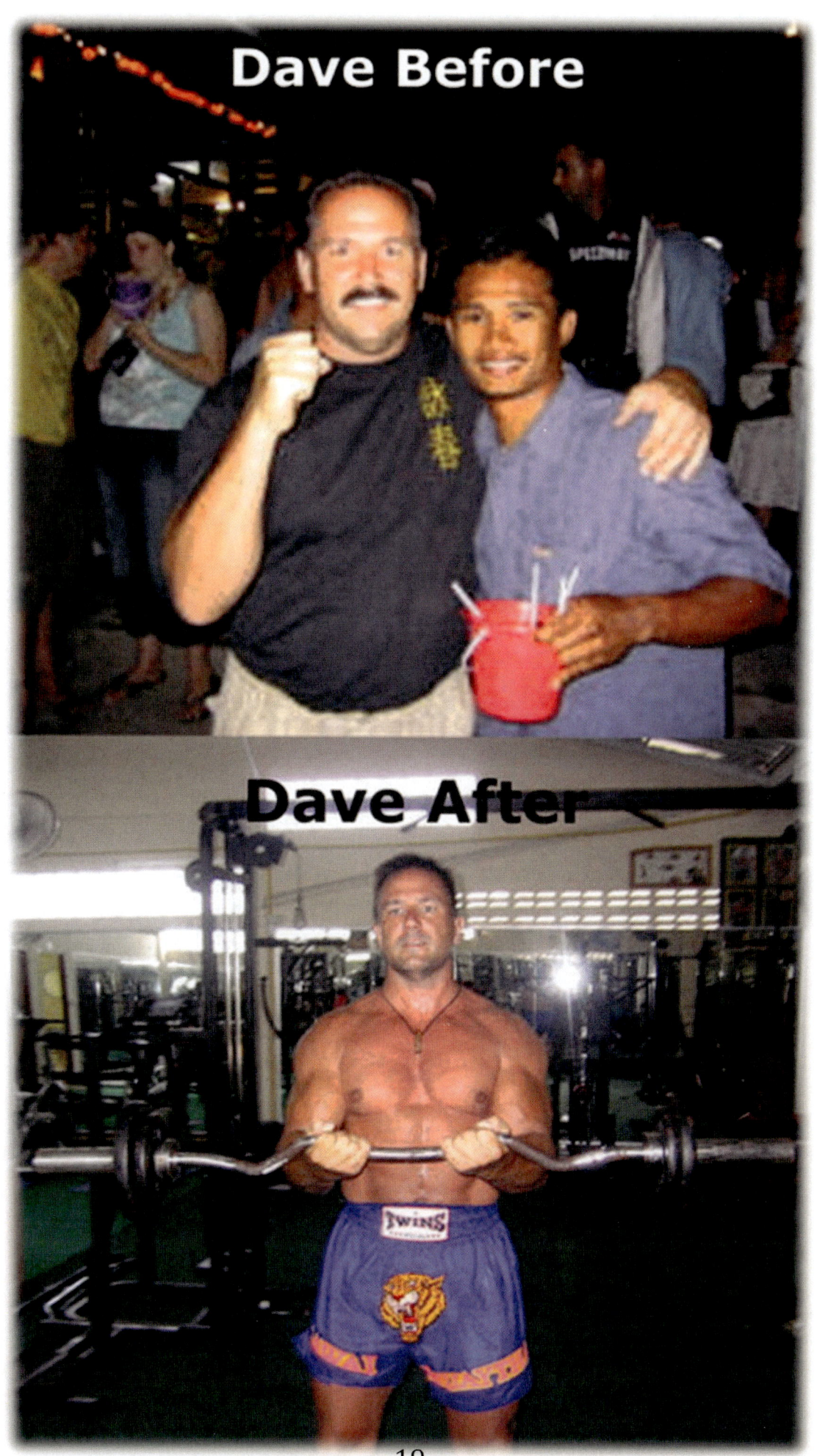

Detox

Detox & Revitalize

We all detox and cleanse for a variety of reasons. Whether it be for weight loss, fatigue, too much food or drink, or like many – just an annual spring cleaning. Whatever your reason is, we're here to assist you. Expect to lose between 12 to 22 pounds in 6 to 10 days. And expect to look and feel better than you have in years!

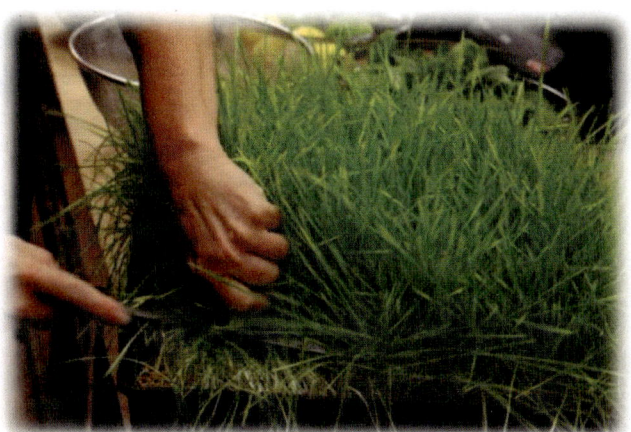
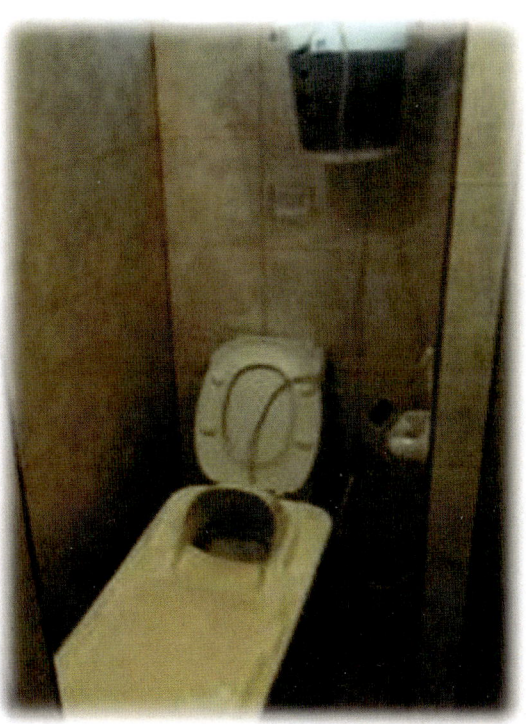
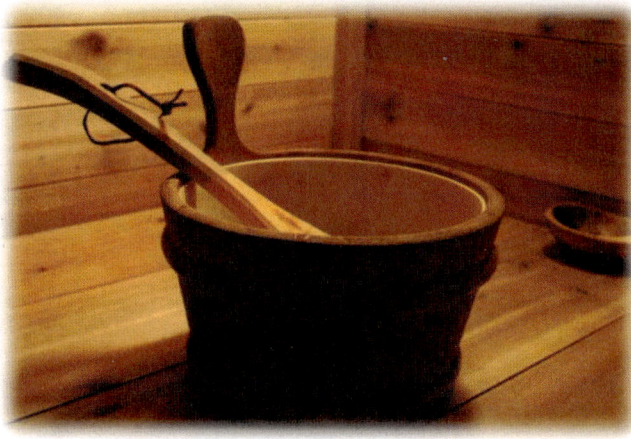
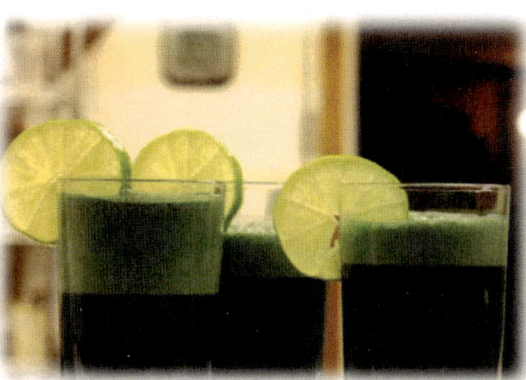

Carrot, Apple & Green

This is tasty! It's a drink we don't normally serve here at the ranch because calories and sugar content are high. If we have a guest coming off of alcohol or sugar, they tend to want this type of drink. As served at DetoxOasis.net.

2	ea	carrots	1	ea	cucumber
2	ea	celery stalks	1	ea	apple
1	handful	spinach (about 2 cups)			

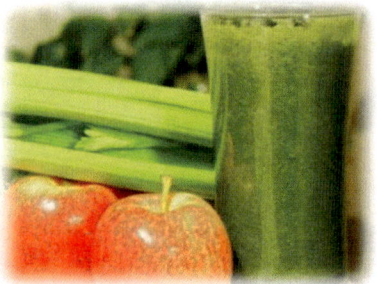

Procedure
1 Blend all ingredients in a Vita-mix or other blender and serve.

Equipment Needed:
1 Vita-mix or other strong blender

Servings: 2

Preparation Time: 5 minutes
Cooking Time:
Total Time: 5 minutes

Nutrition Facts
Serving size: 1/2 of a recipe (14.2 ounces).

Amount Per Serving	
Calories	113.2
Calories From Fat (6%)	6.5
	% Daily Value
Total Fat 0.79g	1%
Saturated Fat 0.11g	<1%
Cholesterol 0mg	0%
Sodium 119.52mg	5%
Potassium 851.6mg	24%
Total Carbohydrates 26.09g	9%
Fiber 6.91g	28%
Sugar 16.38g	
Protein 3.07g	6%
MyPoints 1.53	

Recipe Tips
Anytime you add fruit to something, such as an apple, you add sugar and calories. Most detox centers in the USA won't serve up such a juice. But when I detox, I need more than just green juices on some days. This is a healthy drink any day of the week!

Greatest Detox Vegetable Broth

This is a terrific broth that we use at our ranch that is high in potassium. The veggies are added to a pot of water with herbs and simmered until a rich, delicious broth emerges. Strain and you have 2 quarts broth. Freezes well. At Detox Oasis, we serve just the broth from this recipe for dinner to our detox guests daily at 6pm. Our detox is generally a 6-10 day event followed by healthy foods and fitness. See more on our websites, FitBodyRetreat.com and DetoxOasis.net.

1	lb	celery	1	ea	bay leaf
1-1/2	lb	sweet onions	6	ea	whole black peppercorns
1	lb	carrots (cut into 1" pieces)	1	bunch	fresh parsley, chopped (about 1-1/2 cups)
1	lb	potatoes	1	gallon	water
1/2	lb	turnips, cubed	6	tbsp	Bragg Liquid Aminos
3	ea	garlic cloves			

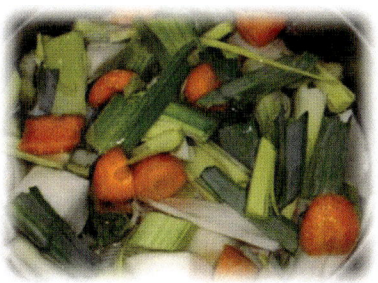

Procedure

1. Toss all veggies in a pot and bring to a boil.
2. Simmer for 1-1/2 to 2 hrs.
3. Cook uncovered until liquid is reduced by half.
4. Pour the broth through a colander, catching the broth in a large bowl or pot. This liquid can be used immediately or stored for later use. We compost the veggies in the pot but you can also eat them. Delicious to eat hot or cold. Don't waste them!
5. Add 1 tbsp of liquid aminos to each bowl.

Servings: 8

Preparation Time: 9 minutes
Cooking Time: 1 hour and 30 minutes
Total Time: 1 hour and 30 minutes

Nutrition Facts

Serving size: 1/8 of a recipe (30.2 ounces).

Amount Per Serving		
Calories		127.85
Calories From Fat (3%)		3.34
		% Daily Value
Total Fat 0.5g		<1%
Saturated Fat 0.08g		<1%
Cholesterol 0mg		0%
Sodium 571.69mg		24%
Potassium 859.22mg		25%
Total Carbohydrates 35.95g		12%
Fiber 5.42g		22%
Sugar 9.85g		
Protein 5.93g		12%
MyPoints 1.8		

Recipe Tips

Stacy from California gave Detox Oasis this recipe. We were missing the potassium component in our detox program. This broth is a "must have" during a detox lasting 1 or more weeks.

Green Algae Drink

We serve this drink 4x/day at the ranch. As served at DetoxOasis.net.

1-1/2	tsp	Spirulina blue green algae powder	6	drops	liquid vanilla stevia
1-1/2	cup	water	1	cup	ice
1	ea	lime, juiced			

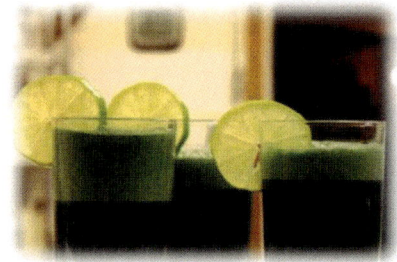

Procedure

1 Mix all together, blend and serve.

Equipment Needed:

1 Vita-mix or other strong blender

Servings: 2

Preparation Time: 4 minutes
Cooking Time:
Total Time: 4 minutes

Nutrition Facts

Serving size: 1/2 of a recipe (20.7 ounces).

Amount Per Serving	
Calories	15.53
Calories From Fat (3%)	0.46
	% Daily Value
Total Fat 0.07g	<1%
Saturated Fat 0.01g	<1%
Cholesterol 0mg	0%
Sodium 8.03mg	<1%
Potassium 35.95mg	1%
Total Carbohydrates 3.91g	1%
Fiber 0.94g	4%
Sugar 0.57g	
Protein 1.21g	2%
MyPoints 0.13	

Recipe Tips

This drink is what I have when I'm fasting or just out of energy. In about 20 minutes, it will regulate your blood sugar, regardless if it's up or down. The reason that I use this drink is it does not cause you nausea like wheat grass can. Wheatgrass is wonderful, but it's very powerful. We train so hard here at our retreat that about 50% of my clients cannot handle the nausea that wheatgrass can produce. So for these clients, it's algae! This recipe was created by my son Rob, and a client of ours, Hap, at one of our Costa Rica retreats.

Green Smoothie & Berries

Refreshing and healthy smoothie. Loaded with minerals, vitamins and taste. As served at DetoxOasis.net.

1	cup	spinach
2	ea	bananas, small
1/2	cup	strawberries (or any berries)
1	ea	orange

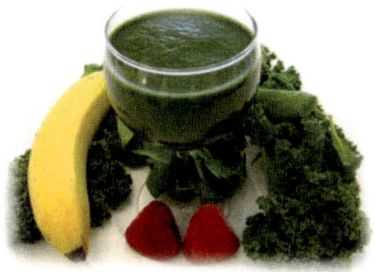

Procedure

1 Put all ingredients in a Vita-mix or other blender and blend until creamy smooth.

Equipment Needed:

1 Vita-mix or other strong blender

Servings: 2

Preparation Time: 5 minutes
Cooking Time: 5 minutes
Total Time: 5 minutes

Nutrition Facts

Serving size: 1/2 of a recipe (8.2 ounces).

Amount Per Serving	
Calories	155.59
Calories From Fat (4%)	5.98
	% Daily Value
Total Fat 0.74g	1%
Saturated Fat 0.16g	<1%
Cholesterol 0mg	0%
Sodium 14.83mg	<1%
Potassium 659.24mg	19%
Total Carbohydrates 38.85g	13%
Fiber 7.29g	29%
Sugar 14.27g	
Protein 2.82g	6%
MyPoints 2.37	

Recipe Tips

If you'd like your smoothie to be even smoother, add an avocado. If sweeter, add mango, pear, coconut, etc.; even a teaspoon of agave. Simple guidelines for any successful smoothie include: anything green - spinach, kale, etc.; any fruit - berries, bananas, peaches, etc.; anything you want - herbs, celery, garlic, sea veggies, etc.

Yes, it's really healthy and pretty tasty. Add a scoop of vanilla protein and it goes from 2 grams to 25 grams of protein! I often add a scoop of protein to my veggie juices simply to reduce the number of items or drinks I consume in a day. Plus, it's faster to only have to clean the blender once.

Green Veggie Juice #1

We serve this drink 2x/day at the ranch. As served at DetoxOasis.net.

1	ea	cucumber	2	ea	celery stalks
2	handfuls	spinach (about 4 cups)	1	dash	cayenne pepper (optional)
1	handful	sprouts (any kind - about 1 cup)			

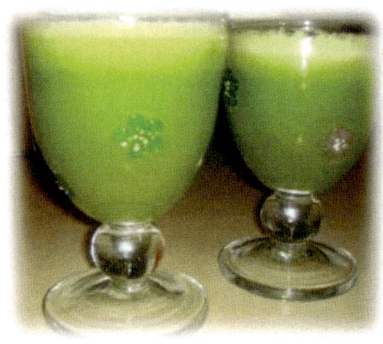

Procedure

1. Mix all ingredients in a Vita-mix blender.
2. Season with cayenne pepper if you'd like to spice it up.
3. Serve and enjoy!

Equipment Needed:

1. Vita-mix or other strong blender

Servings: 1

Preparation Time: 5 minutes
Cooking Time:
Total Time: 5 minutes

Nutrition Facts

Serving size: Entire recipe (21.9 ounces).

Amount Per Serving	
Calories	87.81
Calories From Fat (11%)	9.34
	% Daily Value
Total Fat 1.15g	2%
Saturated Fat 0.16g	<1%
Cholesterol 0mg	0%
Sodium 175.06mg	7%
Potassium 1329.28mg	38%
Total Carbohydrates 14.83g	5%
Fiber 6.3g	25%
Sugar 6.45g	
Protein 6.91g	14%
MyPoints 1.05	

Recipe Tips

Here is a drink I enjoyed at Hippocrates Institute in south Florida. We serve this twice daily during a detox at our fasting and cleansing center, Detox Oasis.

Green Veggie Juice #2

A refreshing juice without a juicer. As served at DetoxOasis.net.

| 1-1/2 | cup | Kale (or spinach) | 6 | cups | water |
| 2 | ea | apples, medium | | | |

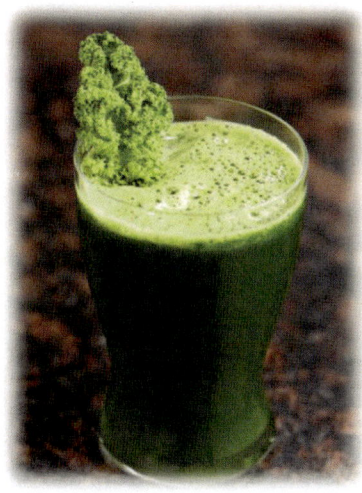

Procedure

1. Blend all ingredients in a Vita-mix or other blender.
2. Pour blended mixture into a nut milk bag.
3. Squeeze mixture over a large bowl and collect the juice.
4. Drink and enjoy!

Equipment Needed:

1. Vita-mix or other strong blender
2. Nut milk bag

Servings: 6

Preparation Time: 5 minutes
Total Time: 5 minutes

Nutrition Facts

Serving size: 1/6 of a recipe (11.1 ounces).

Amount Per Serving	
Calories	39.92
Calories From Fat (4%)	1.76
	% Daily Value
Total Fat 0.22g	<1%
Saturated Fat 0.03g	<1%
Cholesterol 0mg	0%
Sodium 14.92mg	<1%
Potassium 142.16mg	4%
Total Carbohydrates 10.05g	3%
Fiber 1.79g	7%
Sugar 6.3g	
Protein 0.71g	1%
MyPoints 0.46	

Recipe Tips

OK, here is another "Kale Mary, save your life" drink. This drink is so healthy! My only issue with Kale is it does not go through my juicer very well.

Growing Sprouts & Making Rejuvelac

How to grow sprouts at home and make rejuvelac.   As we do at DetoxOasis.net.

2 cups   hard winter wheat (or whatever seed you wish to grow)

4 cups   water

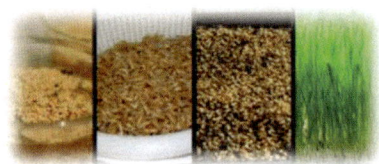

Procedure

1. Cover the seeds with water and soak overnight.
2. Drain the water. The water from the overnight soaked seeds becomes Rejuvelac*
3. Rinse the seeds at least 4x throughout the day. You can't over-rinse, but you can under-rinse.
4. The following day after rinse day, it's time to plant.
5. Put a layer of topsoil in your planting tray, about 1-2" thick.
6. Press the dirt down using another tray so the dirt is compressed.
7. Spread the wheat grass seeds on the dirt, making it thick and heavy, about 1/4" thick. Water heavily.
8. Place an empty tray on the seeds. Then turn off light.
9. Take off the cover tray and water your sprouts daily.
10. Take off the cover tray after they are covered for 2 days and expose them to indirect light such as a fluorescent light. Any light will do. It does not need to be a grow light nor a light directly over the plants. (If it's light enough not to bang your knee on something, it's light enough for the grass.)
11. Maintain a temperature that's above 65 degrees. Harvest after 5-6 days in the dirt. Juice and enjoy!

Servings: 12

Preparation Time: 10 minutes
Cooking Time: 24 hours
Total Time: 24 hours

Nutrition Facts

Serving size: 1/12 of a recipe (3.9 ounces).

Amount Per Serving	
Calories	104.64
Calories From Fat (4%)	4.12
	% Daily Value
Total Fat 0.49g	<1%
Saturated Fat 0.09g	<1%
Cholesterol 0mg	0%
Sodium 3.01mg	<1%
Potassium 116.95mg	3%
Total Carbohydrates 22.78g	8%
Fiber 3.9g	16%
Sugar 0.13g	
Protein 4.04g	8%
MyPoints 1.35	

Recipe Tips

The expert on this is Michael Bergonzi at [Hippocrates Institute](#). Most sprouting books teach you a variety of soak times. Personally, I just soak them all overnight, then do the rinse process, and they turn out fine. My favorite sprout is sunflower sprouts! I know I've said it before, but one thing is certain, if I were told I had just a few months to live, I'd first go on a 100% juice diet. After I cured myself, I'd then go 100% raw, and never make fun of raw foodists again! In my opinion, raw foods can and will cure about any illness the body may encounter.

* Rejuvelac from the soaked seeds is the nasty smelling liquid we use in our alternative cheese recipes.

Liver Flush

See the Detox Protocol at the end of this book for complete instructions. This is our liver flush recipe that we use at the ranch. As served at DetoxOasis.net.

4	cups	water
4	tbsp	Epsom salt
1	ea	grapefruit, juiced
1	pinch	cayenne pepper
1	cup	extra virgin olive oil

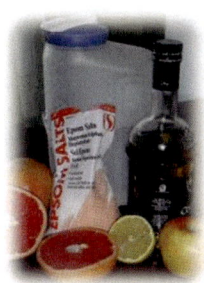

Procedure

Salt Drink
1. Don't eat anything the day of your flush and stop consuming all fluids by 2pm the day of your flush.
2. Mix Epsom salt with water. Pour equal amounts of salt water mixture into 3 individual drinking containers with lids.
3. Label the containers: 6pm, 7pm, and 7am (the next morning) and drink them at the correct times.

Oil Drink
1. Mix the oil and the juice from 1 grapefruit with a pinch of cayenne pepper in a blender or shake well.
2. Label the oil drink 9pm. You'll drink this the day of your flush after your salt drinks.
3. Shake before drinking and drink it at the correct time.

The Next Day
1. Begin drinking plain water again at 9am after your 7am salt drink. Your flush is now complete. If possible get a colonic the day after.

Equipment Needed:
1. Vita-mix or other strong blender

Servings: 1

Preparation Time: 10 minutes
Cooking Time:
Total Time: 10 minutes

Nutrition Facts

Serving size: Entire recipe (58.7 ounces).

Amount Per Serving	
Calories	1991.8
Calories From Fat (95%)	1901.65
	% Daily Value
Total Fat 216.28g	333%
Saturated Fat 29.83g	149%
Cholesterol 0mg	0%
Sodium 32.79mg	1%
Potassium 13.91mg	<1%
Total Carbohydrates 21.06g	7%
Fiber 0.03g	<1%
Sugar 0.01g	
Protein 2.01g	4%
MyPoints 57.85	

Recipe Tips

95% of all my clients drink this at my center. 5% say they are unable to drink it because of religious reasons or some other nonsensical excuse! In my opinion, these drinks taken on day 4 are the graduation dance of any good detox. Without this drink? -- Well, you simply did not finish your detox, nor will you receive the full benefits of your detox.

Psyllium & Bentonite Clay Drink

Our colon cleansing staple here at the Oasis! As served at DetoxOasis.net.

| 1 | tbsp | psyllium husks | 6 | oz | water |
| 1 | tbsp | bentonite clay (liquid) | 1 | sprinkle | cinnamon |

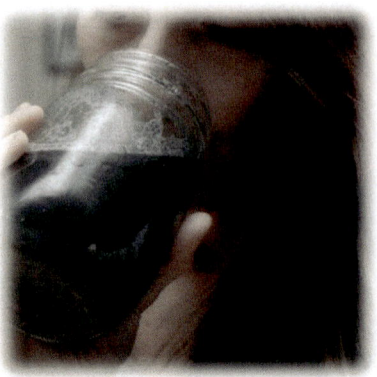

Procedure

1. Mix all ingredients together and drink quickly.
2. Wash glass well immediately!

Servings: 1

Preparation Time: 1 minute
Cooking Time:
Total Time: 1 minute

Nutrition Facts

Serving size: Entire recipe (13.1 ounces).

Amount Per Serving	
Calories	16.7
Calories From Fat (0%)	0
	% Daily Value
Total Fat 0g	0%
Saturated Fat 0g	0%
Cholesterol 0mg	0%
Sodium 5.13mg	<1%
Potassium 2.92mg	<1%
Total Carbohydrates 4.23g	1%
Fiber 0.15g	<1%
Sugar 0.01g	
Protein 0.01g	<1%
MyPoints 0.3	

Recipe Tips

Drink this drink 4x/day during a cleanse. If you are drinking this, you are on your way to a good detox. Yum!

Seaweed Mineral Drink

A bold RAW drink we serve at the ranch. Loaded with vitamins and minerals. This recipe was brought to us by Kat, a friend and occasionally our raw food chef from Bloomington, Indiana. As served at DetoxOasis.net.

1	ea	apple		1	tbsp	kelp
1	ea	orange		1/2	tsp	garlic
3	ea	dates		1/2	ea	banana
2	tbsp	Spirulina blue green algae powder		1	tbsp	agave
2	tbsp	chlorella				

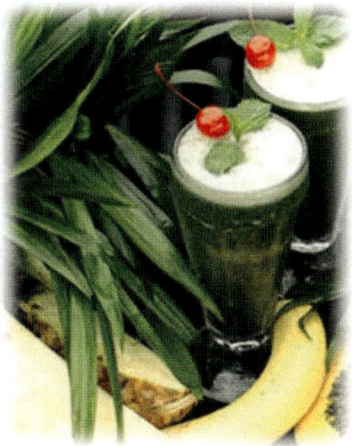

Procedure
1 Place all items in Vita-mix or other blender.
2 Blend well and serve.

Equipment Needed:
1 Vita-mix or other strong blender

Servings: 2

Preparation Time: 5 minutes
Cooking Time:
Total Time: 5 minutes

Nutrition Facts

Serving size: 1/2 of a recipe (20 ounces).

Amount Per Serving	
Calories	239.79
Calories From Fat (2%)	5.44
	% Daily Value
Total Fat 0.56g	<1%
Saturated Fat 0.1g	<1%
Cholesterol 0mg	0%
Sodium 30.59mg	1%
Potassium 445.5mg	13%
Total Carbohydrates 42.94g	14%
Fiber 7.57g	30%
Sugar 20.97g	
Protein 11.38g	23%
MyPoints 4.04	

Recipe Tips

If I was told I only had a few months to live, there are certain foods I would turn to. Just about 100% of them are raw. Raw foods are clean and pure and will heal you, if used correctly. Don't let my occasional negative attitude regarding raw foodists say otherwise. This recipe is one of those, "serious fuel, little fun, high nutrition, save your ass when you are pronounced dying", drinks. Recipe from Kat, friend and client at Spirit Tree Farms in Bloomington, Indiana.

Breakfast

The Oasis Grounds

Environment is important when you do a detox/cleanse from any life event that includes changing or eliminating the consumption of anything you've been doing and now choose to stop – anything from Diet Coke to Starbucks.

Discontinuing or reducing your food, drink, drug or smoke causes discomfort and pain. You must get away from distractions, fast food advertisements, people you love, and the general population itself. The Oasis is about as remote and isolated as you can get. It is here that positive change is made possible and bearable. All of your personal accomplishments that you achieve at the Oasis are private. We live in a toxic society. Take time out for your body and it will reward you beauty, energy and extended life.

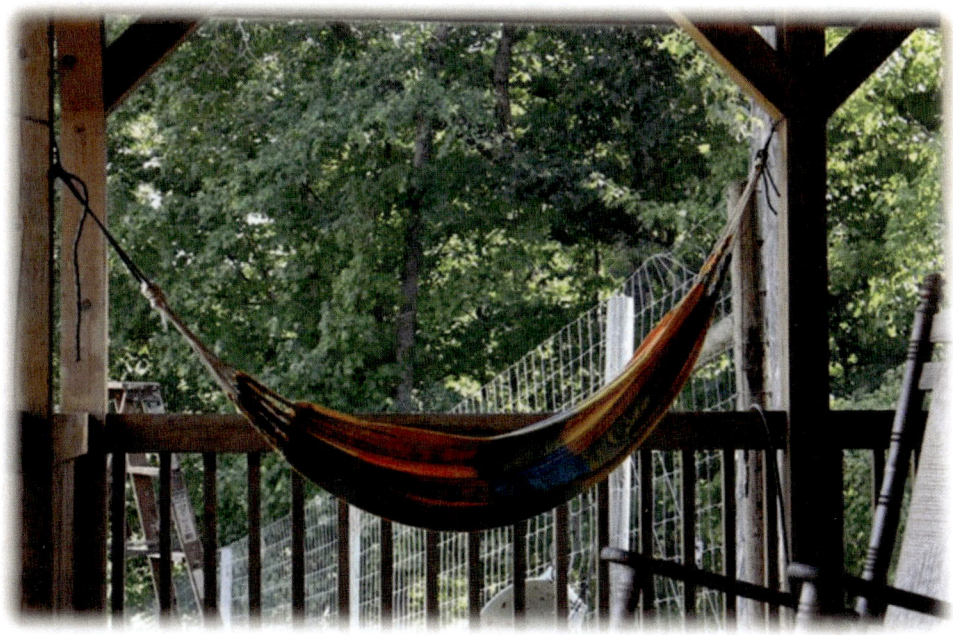

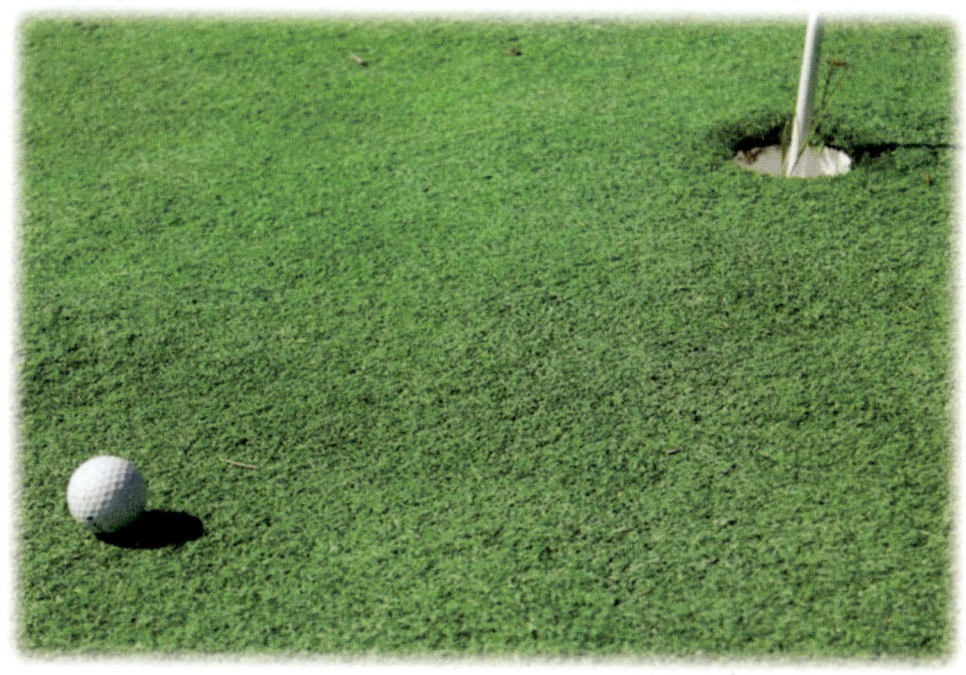

Berries & Yogurt

This is so good! Perfect for that morning when you are not really hungry but know you should eat something good just to get some energy. Your choice of berries - or a combination of them. Strawberries, raspberries, or blueberries. Sprinkled with shaved almonds. As served at FitBodyRetreat.com.

1	cup	vanilla yogurt, fat free	4	tbsp	almonds, raw shaved
1/2	cup	blueberries, fresh (any berry)*			

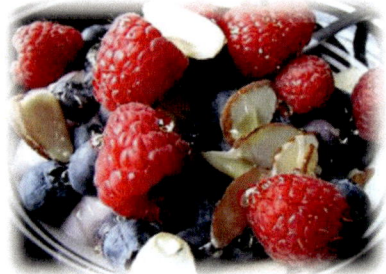

Procedure

1. Pour berries on top of the yogurt.
2. Top with shaved almonds.

Servings: 1

Preparation Time: 5 minutes
Cooking Time:
Total Time: 5 minutes

Nutrition Facts

Serving size: Entire recipe (7.1 ounces).

Amount Per Serving	
Calories	382.13
Calories From Fat (31%)	119.67
	% Daily Value
Total Fat 14.24g	22%
Saturated Fat 0.02g	<1%
Cholesterol 0mg	0%
Sodium 140.74mg	6%
Potassium 56.98mg	2%
Total Carbohydrates 53.72g	18%
Fiber 1.78g	7%
Sugar 7.37g	
Protein 16.55g	33%
MyPoints 8.47	

Recipe Tips

Children can be picky eaters. That is a fact of life. Compensating by feeding them garbage foods because they won't eat the healthy foods you offer them should be a crime that parents need to be held accountable for. When I see a 12 year old 50 pounds overweight, I wonder how a parent could do this to the child they love? Don't they know that diabetes is just around the corner and a lifetime of obesity is their future? If you are a parent, take charge. Do the right thing for your children and give them the best shot at life and health. It's really up to you.

* Calories are pretty close for all the berries.

Breakfast Burritos

High protein and yummy! My goodness -- these are so clean and taste so Mexican! As served at FitBodyRetreat.com.

15	oz	bag black beans (soaked overnight)*
8	ea	egg whites
2	ea	eggs, whole
8	ea	tortilla wrap, low calorie, low carb (10")
8	tbsp	cheddar cheese, shredded, reduced fat
16	oz	pico-de-gallo*
8	ea	lettuce leaves
8	tbsp	refried beans
1	bunch	fresh cilantro

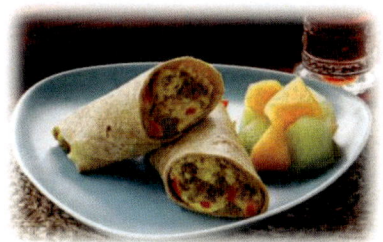

Procedure

1. Add beans to pot of water and simmer for about 1-1/2 hrs.
2. Spray a non-stick pan with zero calorie cooking spray.
3. Scramble eggs in pan.
4. Chop up cilantro in a large bowl.
5. Heat tortillas in a microwave or oven until soft.
6. Lay the tortillas flat and spread about 2 tbsp of refried beans on the tortilla.
7. Spoon as many black beans onto each tortilla as you like.
8. Follow with eggs, cheese, lettuce, cilantro and salsa.
9. Roll the tortillas into burritos.
10. Serve or let cool first.
11. Freeze for reheating and eating another morning.

Servings: 8

Preparation Time: 10 minutes
Cooking Time: 1 hour and 30 minutes
Total Time: 30 minutes

Nutrition Facts

Serving size: 1/8 of a recipe (10.7 ounces).

Amount Per Serving	
Calories	190.18
Calories From Fat (21%)	40.12

	% Daily Value
Total Fat 4.59g	7%
Saturated Fat 0.81g	4%
Cholesterol 48.23mg	16%
Sodium 226.86mg	9%
Potassium 150.3mg	4%
Total Carbohydrates 23.41g	8%
Fiber 0.95g	4%
Sugar 0.48g	
Protein 15.22g	30%
MyPoints 4	

Recipe Tips

Try to get as close to nature as possible. If you plan ahead with your black beans, this dish can be ready in 30 min. If you're in a hurry, you can substitute canned beans, but you may regret it due to sodium content!

* Do not use canned beans as the sodium content triples what the recipe calls for.
* See recipe for Pico-de-Gallo.

Breakfast Quinoa

Nutty cinnamon quinoa - served warm! Use red or white quinoa or combine the two. Use whatever low fat milk you desire - dairy, soy, almond, etc. Also, any berry may be used. Dark honey can replace agave. And use whatever nut you'd like. As served at FitBodyRetreat.com.

1	cup	milk, low fat, 1%
1	cup	water
1	cup	quinoa
2	cups	blackberries, fresh
1/2	tsp	cinnamon
1/3	cup	pecans, chopped, toasted (or whatever nuts are on hand)
4	tsp	agave

Procedure

1. Rinse quinoa well before cooking.
2. Combine milk, water and quinoa in a medium saucepan.*
3. Bring to a boil over high heat.
4. Reduce heat to a medium-low. Cover and simmer 15 min or until most of the liquid is absorbed.
5. Turn off heat and let stand covered 5 min.
6. Stir in blackberries and cinnamon.
7. Transfer to four bowls and top with roasted pecans.
8. Drizzle 1 tsp of agave over each serving.

Servings: 4

Preparation Time: 10 minutes
Cooking Time: 20 minutes
Total Time: 30 minutes

Nutrition Facts

Serving size: 1/4 of a recipe (12.1 ounces).

Amount Per Serving	
Calories	296.49
Calories From Fat (32%)	94.14
	% Daily Value
Total Fat 10.06g	15%
Saturated Fat 1.26g	6%
Cholesterol 3.05mg	1%
Sodium 40.5mg	2%
Potassium 486.61mg	14%
Total Carbohydrates 38.75g	13%
Fiber 7.83g	31%
Sugar 7.05g	
Protein 9.9g	20%
MyPoints 5.97	

Recipe Tips

Watch the serving size here! This is a favorite of mine. Make it up in quantity and freeze it in ¼ cups. Serve warm -- not too hot. Make sure the fruit, agave and nuts go on top after it's already served up and in the bowl.

* While quinoa cooks, roast the pecans in a 350F toaster oven for 5-6 min. or in a dry skillet over medium heat for about 3 min.

Breakfast Tacos

Hot and spicy! High in protein plus good carbs. A good start to the day. As served at FitBodyRetreat.com.

4	oz	ground turkey	1	ea	tomato, medium
1	tbsp	macadamia nut oil	1/4	cup	onion
		Non-stick cooking spray	1/3	cup	cottage cheese, low fat 1%
1	ea	egg, whole			
4	ea	egg whites	1	ea	jalapeno pepper, seeds removed (optional if you like it hot!)
3	tbsp	salsa			
1/4	cup	cilantro			
			3	ea	corn tortillas

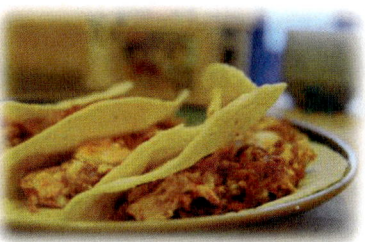

Procedure

1. Cook the turkey in oil in a non-stick pan. Set aside.
2. Scramble the eggs using the non-stick pan and non-stick cooking spray.
3. Place all ingredients into the tortillas in equal amounts.
4. Roll up tortillas and serve.

Servings: 1

Preparation Time: 10 minutes
Cooking Time: 15 minutes
Total Time: 20 minutes

Nutrition Facts

Serving size: Entire recipe (28.3 ounces).

Amount Per Serving	
Calories	714.96
Calories From Fat (38%)	273.37
	% Daily Value
Total Fat 30.9g	48%
Saturated Fat 4.7g	24%
Cholesterol 267.67mg	89%
Sodium 975.4mg	41%
Potassium 1327.63mg	38%
Total Carbohydrates 52.66g	18%
Fiber 7.7g	31%
Sugar 10.16g	
Protein 59.65g	119%
MyPoints 16.07	

Recipe Tips

Give these a go! Healthy stuff to build a lean, sexy body!

Cottage Cheese with Banana & Flax

As served at FitBodyRetreat.com

1/2	cup	cottage cheese, low fat 1%
1	ea	banana, medium
1	tsp	flax seeds, ground
1/2	tsp	agave

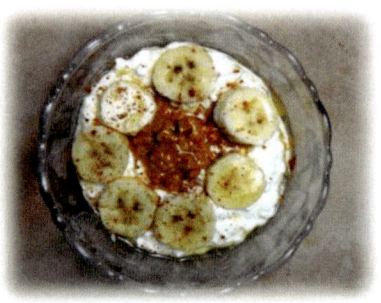

Procedure

1. Slice banana and place the slices over the cottage cheese.
2. Add the ground flax on top.
3. Drizzle agave on top.

Servings: 1

Preparation Time: 5 minutes
Cooking Time:
Total Time: 5 minutes

Nutrition Facts

Serving size: Entire recipe (10 ounces).

Amount Per Serving	
Calories	209.73
Calories From Fat (11%)	23.44
	% Daily Value
Total Fat 2.6g	4%
Saturated Fat 0.95g	5%
Cholesterol 4.52mg	2%
Sodium 465.21mg	19%
Potassium 539.95mg	15%
Total Carbohydrates 30.75g	10%
Fiber 3.75g	15%
Sugar 17.54g	
Protein 15.74g	31%
MyPoints 3.66	

Recipe Tips

For me, this is a snack or a small dish served as a side at lunch. It's a staple with me.

Eggs Easy & Quinoa

Yummy over-easy and high protein! As served at FitBodyRetreat.com.

		Non-stick cooking spray	1	slice	bread, low calorie, toasted (35 cal. max)
2	ea	eggs, whole, large	1	tsp	butter, light, unsalted
1	dash	black pepper (to taste)			
1/4	cup	quinoa, cooked*			
1/2	ea	grapefruit			

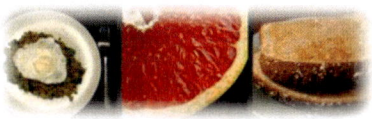

Procedure

1. Spray a non-stick pan with non-stick spray.
2. Crack the eggs open into the pan.
3. Cook the eggs until done. Flip as required.
4. Serve on a plate with a scoop of cooked quinoa, a piece of toast, and 1/2 a grapefruit.

Servings: 1

Preparation Time: 1 minute
Cooking Time: 4 minutes
Total Time: 5 minutes

Nutrition Facts

Serving size: Entire recipe (13.1 ounces).

Amount Per Serving	
Calories	290.4
Calories From Fat (34%)	97.71
	% Daily Value
Total Fat 11.12g	17%
Saturated Fat 3.5g	18%
Cholesterol 373.06mg	124%
Sodium 245.62mg	10%
Potassium 385.64mg	11%
Total Carbohydrates 31.75g	11%
Fiber 3.29g	13%
Sugar 8.85g	
Protein 17.59g	35%
MyPoints 6.08	

Recipe Tips

This reminds me a lot of grits and eggs. If you ever liked those two together, you will like this too!

* See recipe for Quinoa Basic.

Fage 2% Yogurt, Granola & Fresh Fruit

This is a Greek yogurt that is preservative free and loaded with probiotics for a healthy digestive system. Choose from peach, cherry, honey, and strawberry flavors. As served at FitBodyRetreat.com.

1	cup	Fage 2% yogurt	2	tbsp	granola, lite
1/4	cup	blueberries (or any other fruit, honey or agave)			

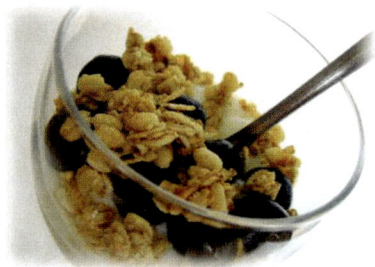

Procedure

1. Open container and pour into bowl.
2. Scoop the fruit onto yogurt.
3. Sprinkle with granola.

Servings: 1

Preparation Time: 5 minutes
Cooking Time: 5 minutes
Total Time: 5 minutes

Nutrition Facts

Serving size: Entire recipe (4.9 ounces).

Amount Per Serving	
Calories	156.59
Calories From Fat (23%)	36.39
	% Daily Value
Total Fat 4.27g	7%
Saturated Fat 0.01g	<1%
Cholesterol 0mg	0%
Sodium 65.37mg	3%
Potassium 28.49mg	<1%
Total Carbohydrates 14.31g	5%
Fiber 0.89g	4%
Sugar 3.69g	
Protein 17.42g	35%
MyPoints 3.31	

Recipe Tips

In my opinion, we lead 3 lives regarding our weight and fitness. 1. Pre goal- where you are today compared to your desired weight or body fat percentage goal 2. Goal- you have reached your desired goal 3. Post goal- you have reached goal but put on some weight. Determine where you are now in your life. Set a goal, stick with it and don't lie to yourself about why you must eat garbage foods when you feel depressed. Take control. Reach your goal and be stronger than the addiction to high carb, high fat foods.

Flaxseed Blueberry Pancakes

Another breakfast served at FitBodyRetreat.com.

1-1/4	cup	whole wheat flour	1-1/3	cup	milk, skim
2/3	cup	flax seeds, ground	1	ea	egg, whole
1	tbsp	cinnamon	1	tsp	vanilla extract
1	tbsp	agave	3/4	cup	blueberries, fresh
2	tsp	baking powder	4	tbsp	pure maple syrup

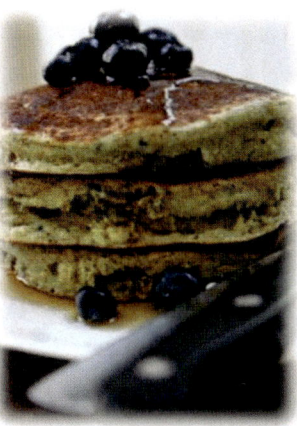

Procedure

1. In a large bowl, mix the whole wheat flour, flaxseed, cinnamon, agave and baking powder; then set aside.
2. In a medium bowl, whisk the skim milk, egg and vanilla.
3. Pour milk mixture into the flour mixture and stir thoroughly.
4. Add blueberries to the mix.
5. Preheat a non-stick pan over medium heat.
6. Spray pan with non-stick spray.
7. Place spoonfuls of batter into the heated pan.
8. Cook as you would any pancakes, just until bubbles appear on the top of each pancake.
9. Flip and cook until a nice light brown, about 1 to 1-1/2 minutes.

Servings: 4

Preparation Time: 15 minutes
Cooking Time: 10 minutes
Total Time: 30 minutes

Nutrition Facts

Serving size: 1/4 of a recipe (8.4 ounces).

Amount Per Serving	
Calories	405.6
Calories From Fat (29%)	117.5
	% Daily Value
Total Fat 13.32g	20%
Saturated Fat 1.51g	8%
Cholesterol 46.5mg	16%
Sodium 279.94mg	12%
Potassium 437.69mg	13%
Total Carbohydrates 58.31g	19%
Fiber 12.77g	51%
Sugar 15.63g	
Protein 14.54g	29%
MyPoints 8.42	

Recipe Tips

Why cheat one day a week? The body is a fat storing device and it's damn good at it. To speed up the body's calorie burn rate, you've got to trick it each week. That trick is to eat some high carb and high fat foods! Make your body think all is well with a good slice of pizza, and it quickly turns off its fat storing mechanism. The down side of eating these carbs and fat is that you're activating your carb desires, meaning you are going to crave carbs again for the next two or three days. And don't think that the fish cake recipe in here qualifies for a good cheat!

French Toast

Delicious! Top with sliced strawberries or blueberries. As served at FitBodyRetreat.com.

		Non-stick cooking spray	1	tsp	cinnamon
4	ea	egg whites	8	slices	bread, low calorie (35 cal. max)
1	ea	egg, whole	4	tbsp	agave
12	tbsp	protein powder, vanilla (lite)	1	cup	blueberries, fresh (or any berry)

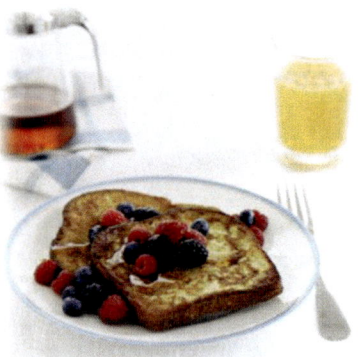

Procedure

1. Whisk together eggs, protein powder and cinnamon in a large bowl.
2. Spray non-stick spray onto a non-stick frying pan over medium heat.
3. Dunk each slice of bread in egg mixture, soaking both sides.
4. Place in pan and cook on both sides until golden brown, about 3-4 min per side.
5. Serve hot and top with agave, about 1/2 tbsp per slice, and berries.

Servings: 4

Preparation Time: 10 minutes
Cooking Time: 10 minutes
Total Time: 20 minutes

Nutrition Facts

Serving size: 1/4 of a recipe (31.7 ounces).

Amount Per Serving	
Calories	336.44
Calories From Fat (18%)	61.22
	% Daily Value
Total Fat 5.88g	9%
Saturated Fat 0.4g	2%
Cholesterol 46.5mg	16%
Sodium 395.13mg	16%
Potassium 102.98mg	3%
Total Carbohydrates 30.47g	10%
Fiber 1.23g	5%
Sugar 3.98g	
Protein 29.01g	58%
MyPoints 6.97	

Recipe Tips

29 grams of protein in French Toast is what I call a good breakfast! The calories are fine and the taste is amazing! Here is one that the kids don't even know is healthy!

Fresh Tomato Parmesan Scramble

This simple egg scramble idea features parmesan cheese and tomatoes seasoned with black pepper and garlic salt. As served at FitBodyRetreat.com.

		Non-stick cooking spray	1	dash	black pepper (to taste)
4	ea	egg whites	2	tsp	water
1	ea	egg, whole	1	tsp	parmesan cheese, grated
1	ea	tomato, small, chopped			
1	dash	garlic powder (to taste)	1/2	cup	cottage cheese, low fat 1%

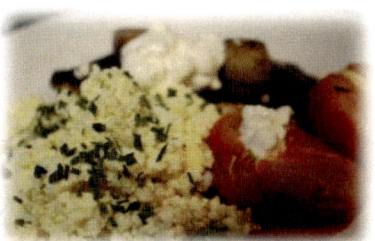

Procedure

1. Prepare a skillet with non-stick cooking spray and place over medium heat.
2. Put half of the chopped tomatoes and the amount of garlic you want in the skillet and season with black pepper.
3. Whisk the eggs, water and parmesan cheese together in a small bowl.
4. Add to skillet.
5. Cook until eggs are set, but still slightly moist, about 5 min.
6. Top with cottage cheese and the remaining tomatoes.

Servings: 1

Preparation Time: 5 minutes
Cooking Time: 5 minutes
Total Time: 10 minutes

Nutrition Facts

Serving size: Entire recipe (14.1 ounces).

Amount Per Serving	
Calories	247.07
Calories From Fat (26%)	63.09
	% Daily Value
Total Fat 6.8g	10%
Saturated Fat 2.61g	13%
Cholesterol 191.99mg	64%
Sodium 782.06mg	33%
Potassium 606.47mg	17%
Total Carbohydrates 8.28g	3%
Fiber 1.14g	5%
Sugar 6.62g	
Protein 36.34g	73%
MyPoints 5.28	

Recipe Tips

A few thoughts on endless cardio -- many of us play "chase the rat on the treadmill". Many people do endless hours of cardio to burn calories. It's difficult to win at that game. I prefer to teach my clients how to make their body do the fat burning work for them. My method is to change and actually increase your body's daily burn rate or metabolism. You can increase your resting burn rate by 300 calories a day by simply adding new lean muscle. Then you can let your new and increased burn rate do the work! And if you add cardio to the mix, it'll become an even more powerful calorie burning combination. Eat foods like this dish combined with strength training, and you are well on your way to a sexy you!

High Protein Oatmeal

Oatmeal porridge with protein powder. Another breakfast served at FitBodyRetreat.com.

4-1/5	cups	water	1	cup	blueberries, fresh*
2	cups	rolled oats	1/4	cup	almonds, raw shaved
1	tbsp	Bragg Liquid Aminos	1	pinch	cinnamon
4	scoops	protein powder			

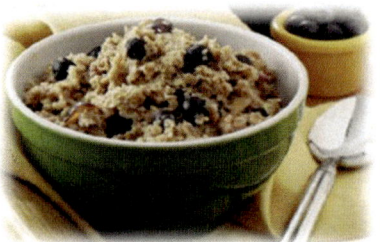

Procedure

1. In a medium saucepan, heat water to boiling. Reduce heat to low; stir in oats and liquid aminos. Cook until oats have thickened, about 5 minutes.
2. Transfer equal amounts of cooked oats to 4 bowls.
3. Stir 1 scoop of protein powder into each bowl.
4. Sprinkle cinnamon on top of each bowl.
5. Add about 1/4 cup of berries to each bowl.
6. Add about 2 tbsp of shaved almonds to each bowl.
7. Serve hot.

Servings: 4

Preparation Time: 5 minutes
Cooking Time: 10 minutes
Total Time: 15 minutes

Nutrition Facts

Serving size: 1/4 of a recipe (13.2 ounces).

Amount Per Serving	
Calories	343.34
Calories From Fat (23%)	79.07
	% Daily Value
Total Fat 9.12g	14%
Saturated Fat 0.01g	<1%
Cholesterol 0mg	0%
Sodium 177.84mg	7%
Potassium 30.71mg	<1%
Total Carbohydrates 37.81g	13%
Fiber 0.91g	4%
Sugar 3.61g	
Protein 30.77g	62%
MyPoints 7.44	

Recipe Tips

Add high calorie protein if you're not trying to shed pounds. Be careful not to add too many toppings such as bananas, as they add calories. Here is how I make it for myself in a jiffy: boil 1 cup of water, then place 1/2 cup of oats in a bowl. Mix together, cover, and go take my shower. By the time I'm dressed and ready, the oats are done. I then mix in 1 scoop of protein powder, and add fresh fruit and almonds. It takes very little time!

High Protein Pancakes

High protein pancakes. As served at FitBodyRetreat.com.

1/2	cup	egg whites
1/2	cup	oats
1/2	cup	cottage cheese, low fat 1%
1/8	tsp	baking powder
1/2	cup	blueberries, frozen (warmed as a topping)
1	drop	liquid stevia (or agave - both optional)
		Non-stick cooking spray

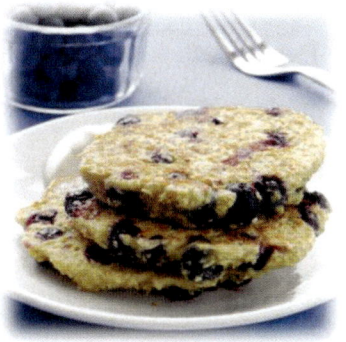

Procedure

1. Mix first 4 ingredients together until smooth. If you use a blender, make sure you put wet ingredients in first.
2. Check to see if pan is hot enough by splashing some water onto it. If it sizzles, it's hot enough.
3. Spray a heated griddle or non-stick pan with non-stick cooking spray and pour approximately 1/4 cup of the batter for each pancake onto it.
4. When pancake bubbles, flip and cook the other side.
5. Top with frozen berries, warmed and sliced and poured over the top with their juices.

Servings: 2

Preparation Time: 15 minutes
Cooking Time: 5 minutes
Total Time: 20 minutes

Nutrition Facts

Serving size: 1/2 of a recipe (10.3 ounces).

Amount Per Serving	
Calories	241.98
Calories From Fat (13%)	30.78
	% Daily Value
Total Fat 3.43g	5%
Saturated Fat 0.85g	4%
Cholesterol 2.26mg	<1%
Sodium 362.54mg	15%
Potassium 338.78mg	10%
Total Carbohydrates 32.75g	11%
Fiber 5.67g	23%
Sugar 1.97g	
Protein 20.21g	40%
MyPoints 4.33	

Recipe Tips

To hire a personal trainer or not? -- For most people, a workout on their own is generally no more than maintenance. Most people who train on their own, train at 40-50% intensity. If you work out with a motivated friend, you may hit 60-70% intensity because you're chitchatting with each other, etc. However, when you train with a professional personal trainer, you can easily hit a workout intensity of 90-100%. So, the simple math tells us that a trainer will get you to your personal fitness goal about 2 times faster than if working out alone. However, if your food/fuel is not in order, you are wasting your time and your money on the trainer. Get your food in order first, then hire a trainer to help accelerate your success!

* You can use any type of berry and substitute frozen for fresh berries. You can also use stevia or agave to taste.

Oaties & Scramble / Pico-de-Gallo

As served at FitBodyRetreat.com.

1	cup	oatmeal, prepared steel cut
2	tsp	agave
1/4	tsp	cinnamon
1	ea	egg, whole
1	ea	egg white
1/2	tsp	macadamia nut oil
1	tsp	pico-de-gallo*
1/2	ea	pear

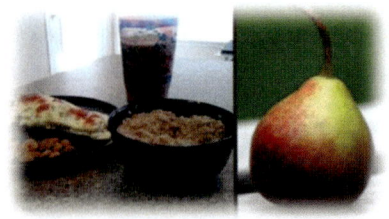

Procedure

1. Prepare oats according to package.
2. Stir agave and cinnamon into oatmeal.
3. Mix egg and egg whites.
4. Heat oil in pan on medium heat.
5. Pour in egg mix and scramble with pico-de-gallo.
6. Serve with 1/2 pear on the side.

Servings: 1

Preparation Time: 5 minutes
Cooking Time: 5 minutes
Total Time: 10 minutes

Nutrition Facts

Serving size: Entire recipe (18 ounces).

Amount Per Serving	
Calories	502.93
Calories From Fat (25%)	127.88
	% Daily Value
Total Fat 13.26g	20%
Saturated Fat 1.57g	8%
Cholesterol 186mg	62%
Sodium 158.73mg	7%
Potassium 232.15mg	7%
Total Carbohydrates 67.22g	22%
Fiber 3.1g	12%
Sugar 9.16g	
Protein 20.28g	41%
MyPoints 10.54	

Recipe Tips

Here is another great oatmeal dish. Breakfast can be fast and high protein! Either have oatmeal with a scoop of protein, ¼ cup of berries, and a few shaved almonds thrown on top; or have what I personally eat for breakfast -- a 5:1 ratio egg omelet with any meat, vegetable and bean that's left over from dinner the night before. I keep it quick and simple and with high protein. We're talking about calories, protein and fuel here. Eat well! 80% of your look depends upon it!

* See recipe for Pico-de-Gallo

Protein Omelet

Another great breakfast. As served at FitBodyRetreat.com.

		Non-stick cooking spray	1/4	ea	red pepper, chopped
1	ea	egg, whole*	2	tbsp	cheese, low fat (or fat free)
4	ea	egg whites*	1/4	ea	yellow bell pepper chopped
1/4	tsp	Bragg Liquid Aminos			
1/8	cup	green onion, chopped	1	cup	cheddar cheese, low fat, shredded
2	oz	chicken, cooked (or turkey)	1/4	cup	black beans, fresh, cooked
1/8	tsp	black pepper	1/2	ea	tomato, medium, chopped

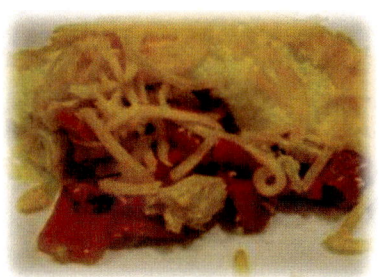

Procedure

1. Spray a non-stick skillet with non-stick cooking spray.*
2. In a bowl, mix eggs with liquid aminos.
3. Pour 1/2 of egg mixture into skillet.
4. As eggs set, lift skillet letting uncooked portions flow underneath.
5. When eggs are set, sprinkle 1/2 of each ingredient in the middle - leaving remaining 1/2 for second omelet.
6. Using spatula, fold it up like a crepe while still in pan.
7. Cover and let stand for 1-2 min or until cheese is melted.
8. Repeat for second omelet.
9. Top with cooked black beans.

Servings: 2

Preparation Time: 5 minutes
Cooking Time: 5 minutes
Total Time: 15 minutes

Nutrition Facts

Serving size: 1/2 of a recipe (11.3 ounces).

Amount Per Serving	
Calories	263.74
Calories From Fat (30%)	79.55
	% Daily Value
Total Fat 8.67g	13%
Saturated Fat 4.03g	20%
Cholesterol 121.3mg	40%
Sodium 578.93mg	24%
Potassium 473.92mg	14%
Total Carbohydrates 10.98g	4%
Fiber 2.98g	12%
Sugar 2.62g	
Protein 34.19g	68%
MyPoints 5.4	

Recipe Tips

If it's not oatmeal for my breakfast, it's an egg white omelet. I'm a creature of habit. Plus these items are so fast and so easy! I can make this omelet in less than 7 minutes.

* If you're in a hurry, use Egg Beaters. You can shave off a few minutes doing it this way.
* I use a large 14" skillet so the egg spreads out like a think crepe. It cooks faster and rolls up easier.

Scrambled Eggs with Cottage Cheese

A client/friend in Hong Kong gave me this recipe. As served at FitBodyRetreat.com.

4	ea	egg whites
1	ea	egg, whole
1	tsp	chives
1	tsp	Bragg Liquid Aminos
1/2	cup	low fat cottage cheese, 1%
1/2	ea	tomato, diced
1	slice	bread, low calorie, toasted (35 cal. max)

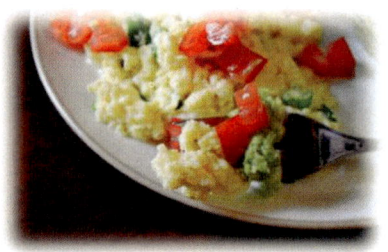

Procedure

1. Scramble the eggs with the chives and liquid aminos in a non-stick pan.
2. Place the cottage cheese and diced tomatoes on top of the eggs.
3. Serve with a slice of toast.

Servings: 1

Preparation Time: 5 minutes
Cooking Time: 5 minutes
Total Time: 10 minutes

Nutrition Facts

Serving size: Entire recipe (13.1 ounces).

Amount Per Serving	
Calories	269.79
Calories From Fat (21%)	56.33
	% Daily Value
Total Fat 6.28g	10%
Saturated Fat 2.31g	12%
Cholesterol 190.52mg	64%
Sodium 1014.96mg	42%
Potassium 547.03mg	16%
Total Carbohydrates 15.08g	5%
Fiber 0.84g	3%
Sugar 6g	
Protein 38.47g	77%
MyPoints 5.75	

Recipe Tips

I spent 14 days detoxing and training at the Oasis center with a client, Rod, from Hong Kong. After the detox, he brought me to his home where I stayed for a month to continue our fitness and foods program with one-on-one personal attention. I thought I was going to teach his two personal chefs how to cook. These gals were experts! Rod taught me this breakfast dish. It's one of my favorite breakfast dishes of all time. I'd put Rod's last name in this book but he's funny that way. Strange – he's been in magazines all of his life. What's the big deal about a silly cookbook, mate!

Scrambled Eggs with Feta & Veggie

As served at FitBodyRetreat.com.

4	ea	egg whites		1/2	oz	Feta cheese crumbled
1	ea	eggs, whole		1	slice	bread, multigrain, toasted
1	tsp	macadamia nut oil				
1	cup	mushrooms, sliced		1	tsp	butter, light, unsalted
1/2	cup	tomato, diced		1	ea	apple, medium

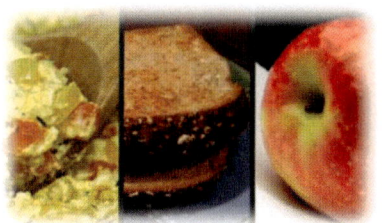

Procedure

1. Heat oil in a non-stick skillet.
2. Sauté the mushrooms and set aside.
3. Mix the egg and egg whites together and scramble until cooked.
4. Stir in diced tomato, mushrooms and feta cheese.
5. Serve with toast and an apple on the side.

Servings: 1

Preparation Time: 5 minutes
Cooking Time: 10 minutes
Total Time: 20 minutes

Nutrition Facts

Serving size: Entire recipe (22.1 ounces).

Amount Per Serving	
Calories	413.46
Calories From Fat (32%)	130.96
	% Daily Value
Total Fat 14.96g	23%
Saturated Fat 4.14g	21%
Cholesterol 199.68mg	67%
Sodium 622.01mg	26%
Potassium 962.51mg	28%
Total Carbohydrates 42.6g	14%
Fiber 5.35g	21%
Sugar 20.32g	
Protein 30.01g	60%
MyPoints 8.72	

Recipe Tips

I'll say this about feta -- add it to almost anything and you have just improved that dish!

Scrambled Eggs with Goat Cheese & Red Peppers

As served at FitBodyRetreat.com.

1/2	tsp	macadamia nut oil	1/8	tsp	black pepper
1/2	ea	red pepper, medium, sliced	1	tsp	Bragg Liquid Aminos
1	ea	egg, whole	1	slice	bread, multigrain, toasted
2	ea	egg whites	1	tsp	jam or jelly, low calorie
1/2	oz	goat cheese, crumbled	1	cup	blackberries (or any berries)

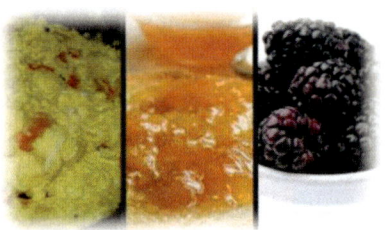

Procedure

1. Heat oil in a non-stick skillet.
2. Add red pepper and sauté.
3. Remove red pepper from pan and set aside.
4. Mix egg and egg whites together.
5. Pour into skillet and scramble.
6. Add the red pepper and goat cheese to pan.
7. Mix all ingredients together.
8. Add black pepper and squirt of liquid aminos.
9. Serve with berries and toast on side.

Servings: 1

Preparation Time: 5 minutes
Cooking Time: 5 minutes
Total Time: 15 minutes

Nutrition Facts

Serving size: Entire recipe (16.3 ounces).

Amount Per Serving	
Calories	355.09
Calories From Fat (33%)	117.46
	% Daily Value
Total Fat 13.37g	21%
Saturated Fat 4.53g	23%
Cholesterol 197.2mg	66%
Sodium 579.41mg	24%
Potassium 594.59mg	17%
Total Carbohydrates 37.47g	12%
Fiber 9.27g	37%
Sugar 13.93g	
Protein 23.39g	47%
MyPoints 7.42	

Recipe Tips

It seems that the Canadians and Europeans that attend my center are keener on goat cheese. I'm no expert on this stuff, but it's really good. If you have some good goat cheese recipes, send them to me if you wish. One thing I really enjoy about this business is the interesting people I meet and the knowledge they share with me.

Beverages & Smoothies

The Oasis Kitchen

The personal trainer of the future will be equally skilled in the kitchen as in the gym. The real and immediate changes to your body happen in the kitchen with the foods you purchase, prepare and consume. The gym time then fine-tunes, tones and sexifies your shape.

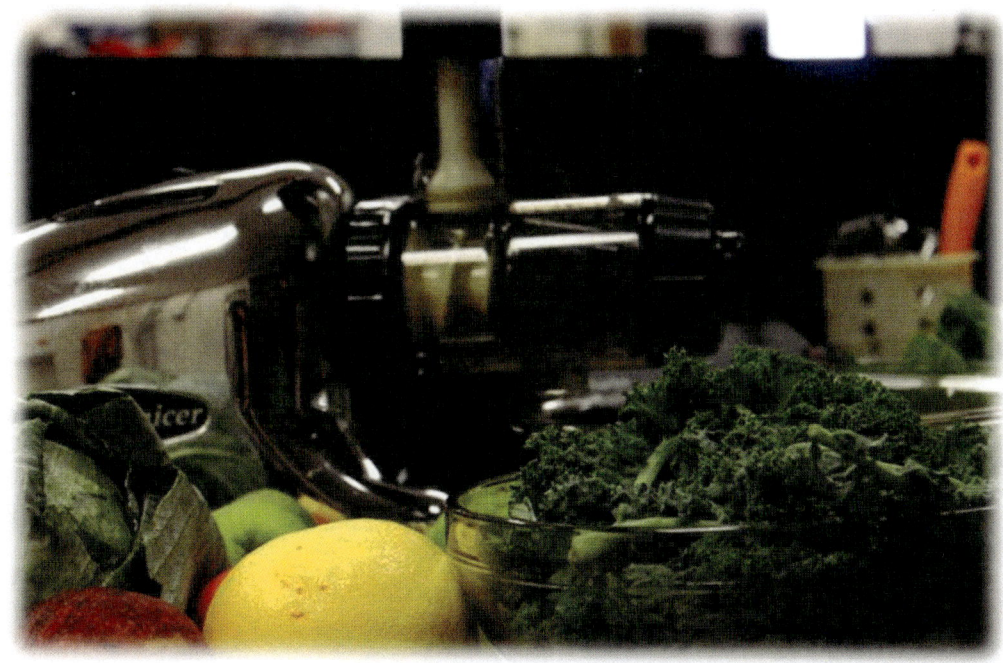

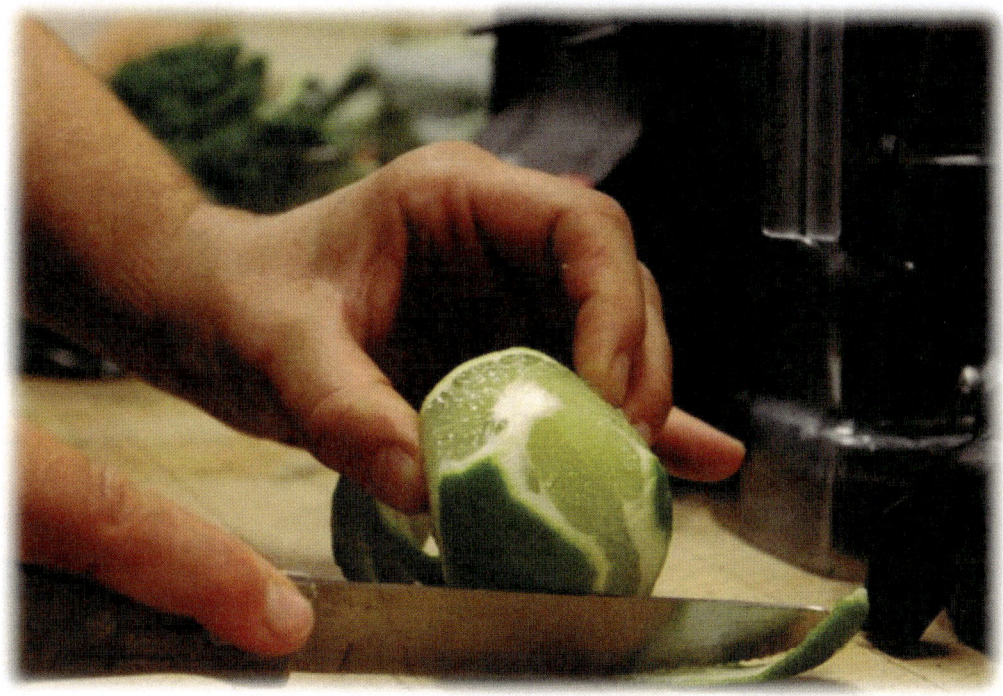

Almond Nut Milk

A fresh healthy drink. As served at DetoxOasis.net.

- 1 cup almonds (soaked overnight)
- 3 cups water
- 1 tsp agave (or 4 drops liquid stevia for less calories)

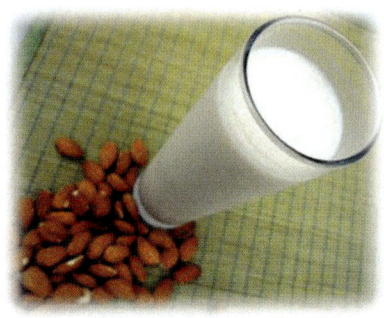

Procedure

10. Soak almonds overnight. Most other nuts take only an hour of soaking.
11. Blend almonds and stevia with water in a Vita-mix or other blender until smooth.
12. Serve.

Equipment Needed:

1. Vita-mix or other strong blender

Servings: 1

Preparation Time: 5 minutes
Cooking Time:
Total Time: 5 minutes

Nutrition Facts

Serving size: Entire recipe (33.7 ounces).

Amount Per Serving	
Calories	842.25
Calories From Fat (72%)	607.81
	% Daily Value
Total Fat 70.67g	109%
Saturated Fat 5.34g	27%
Cholesterol 0mg	0%
Sodium 31.76mg	1%
Potassium 1015.26mg	29%
Total Carbohydrates 30.99g	10%
Fiber 17.45g	70%
Sugar 5.56g	
Protein 30.34g	61%
MyPoints 21.93	

Recipe Tips

Rather than boil your quinoa in just water, try using almond milk, it makes the quinoa really tasty!

Carrot, Apple & Green

This is tasty! It's a drink we don't normally serve here at the ranch because calories and sugar content are high. If we have a guest coming off of alcohol or sugar, they tend to want this type of drink. As served at DetoxOasis.net.

2	ea	carrots	1	ea	cucumber
2	ea	celery stalks	1	ea	apple
1	handful	spinach (about 2 cups)			

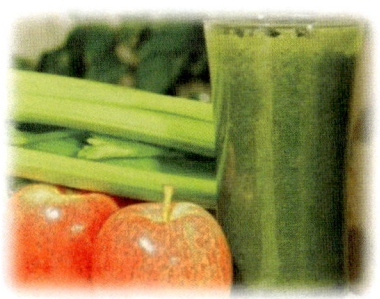

Procedure
1 Blend all ingredients in a Vita-mix or other blender and serve.

Equipment Needed:
1 Vita-mix or other strong blender

Servings: 2

Preparation Time: 5 minutes
Cooking Time:
Total Time: 5 minutes

Nutrition Facts

Serving size: 1/2 of a recipe (14.2 ounces).

Amount Per Serving	
Calories	113.2
Calories From Fat (6%)	6.5
	% Daily Value
Total Fat 0.79g	1%
Saturated Fat 0.11g	<1%
Cholesterol 0mg	0%
Sodium 119.52mg	5%
Potassium 851.6mg	24%
Total Carbohydrates 26.09g	9%
Fiber 6.91g	28%
Sugar 16.38g	
Protein 3.07g	6%
MyPoints 1.53	

Recipe Tips

Anytime you add fruit to something, such as an apple, you add sugar and calories. Most detox centers in the USA won't serve up such a juice. But when I detox, I need more than just green juices on some days. This is a healthy drink any day of the week!

Cocoa Almond Drink

A nice cocoa drink all will enjoy. As served at DetoxOasis.net.

3/4	cup	almond milk	10	drops	liquid vanilla stevia
1	tsp	cocoa powder	2	tsp	extra virgin coconut oil (liquefied*)
1	tsp	agave			

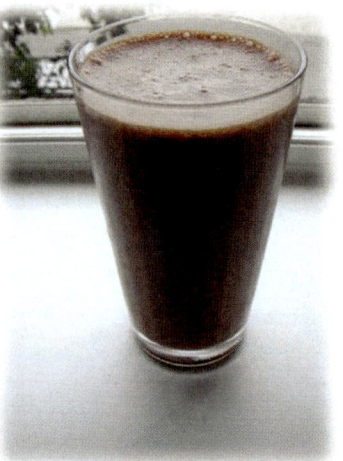

Procedure
1. Blend almond milk, cocoa, agave and stevia in Vita-mix or other blender.
2. Add the coconut oil and blend until smooth and creamy.

Equipment Needed:
1. Vita-mix or other strong blender

Servings: 1

Preparation Time: 5 minutes
Cooking Time:
Total Time: 5 minutes

Nutrition Facts
Serving size: Entire recipe (81.5 ounces).

Amount Per Serving	
Calories	159.84
Calories From Fat (84%)	134.18
	% Daily Value
Total Fat 9.74g	15%
Saturated Fat 0.44g	2%
Cholesterol 0mg	0%
Sodium 118.34mg	5%
Potassium 82.3mg	2%
Total Carbohydrates 3.13g	1%
Fiber 1.79g	7%
Sugar 0.09g	
Protein 1.06g	2%
MyPoints 3.65	

Recipe Tips
One of those raw foodie "rite of passage" drinks.

* Coconut oil must be in liquid form to blend properly.

Green Algae Drink

We serve this drink 4x/day at the ranch. As served at DetoxOasis.net.

1-1/2	tsp	Spirulina blue green algae powder	6	drops	liquid vanilla stevia
1-1/2	cup	water	1	cup	ice
1	ea	lime, juiced			

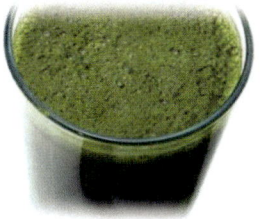

Procedure
1 Mix all together, blend and serve.

Equipment Needed:
1 Vita-mix or other strong blender

Servings: 2

Preparation Time: 4 minutes
Cooking Time:
Total Time: 4 minutes

Nutrition Facts

Serving size: 1/2 of a recipe (20.7 ounces).

Amount Per Serving	
Calories	15.53
Calories From Fat (3%)	0.46
	% Daily Value
Total Fat 0.07g	<1%
Saturated Fat 0.01g	<1%
Cholesterol 0mg	0%
Sodium 8.03mg	<1%
Potassium 35.95mg	1%
Total Carbohydrates 3.91g	1%
Fiber 0.94g	4%
Sugar 0.57g	
Protein 1.21g	2%
MyPoints 0.13	

Recipe Tips

This drink is what I have when I'm fasting or just out of energy. In about 20 minutes, it will regulate your blood sugar, regardless if it's up or down. The reason that I use this drink is it does not cause you nausea like wheat grass can. Wheatgrass is wonderful, but it's very powerful. We train so hard here at our retreat that about 50% of my clients cannot handle the nausea that wheatgrass can produce. So for these clients, it's algae! This recipe was created by my son Rob, and a client of ours, Hap, at one of our Costa Rica retreats.

Green Smoothie & Berries

Refreshing and healthy smoothie. Loaded with minerals, vitamins and taste. As served at DetoxOasis.net.

1	cup	spinach
2	ea	bananas, small
1/2	cup	strawberries (or any berries)
1	ea	orange

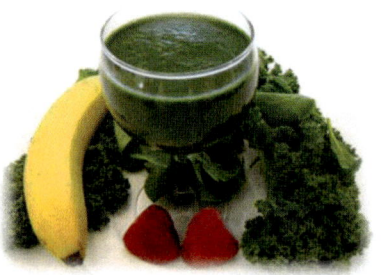

Procedure
1. Put all ingredients in a Vita-mix or other blender and blend until creamy smooth.

Equipment Needed:
1. Vita-mix or other strong blender

Servings: 2

Preparation Time: 5 minutes
Cooking Time: 5 minutes
Total Time: 5 minutes

Nutrition Facts

Serving size: 1/2 of a recipe (8.2 ounces).

Amount Per Serving	
Calories	155.59
Calories From Fat (4%)	5.98
	% Daily Value
Total Fat 0.74g	1%
Saturated Fat 0.16g	<1%
Cholesterol 0mg	0%
Sodium 14.83mg	<1%
Potassium 659.24mg	19%
Total Carbohydrates 38.85g	13%
Fiber 7.29g	29%
Sugar 14.27g	
Protein 2.82g	6%
MyPoints 2.37	

Recipe Tips

If you'd like your smoothie to be even smoother, add an avocado. If sweeter, add mango, pear, coconut, etc.; even a teaspoon of agave. Simple guidelines for any successful smoothie include: anything green - spinach, kale, etc.; any fruit - berries, bananas, peaches, etc.; anything you want - herbs, celery, garlic, sea veggies, etc.

Yes, it's really healthy and pretty tasty. Add a scoop of vanilla protein and it goes from 2 grams to 25 grams of protein! I often add a scoop of protein to my veggie juices simply to reduce the number of items or drinks I consume in a day. Plus, it's faster to only have to clean the blender once.

Green Veggie Juice #1

We serve this drink 2x/day at the ranch. As served at DetoxOasis.net.

1	ea	cucumber
2	handfuls	spinach (about 4 cups)
1	handful	sprouts (any kind - about 1 cup)
2	ea	celery stalks
1	dash	cayenne pepper (optional)

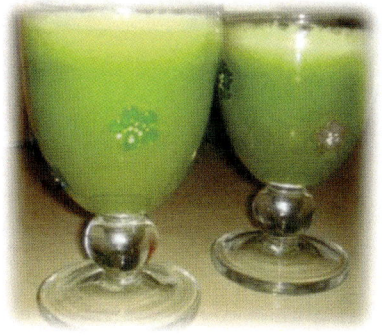

Procedure

1 Mix all ingredients in a Vita-mix blender.
2 Season with cayenne pepper if you'd like to spice it up.
3 Serve and enjoy!

Equipment Needed:

1 Vita-mix or other strong blender

Servings: 1

Preparation Time: 5 minutes
Cooking Time:
Total Time: 5 minutes

Nutrition Facts

Serving size: Entire recipe (21.9 ounces).

Amount Per Serving	
Calories	87.81
Calories From Fat (11%)	9.34
	% Daily Value
Total Fat 1.15g	2%
Saturated Fat 0.16g	<1%
Cholesterol 0mg	0%
Sodium 175.06mg	7%
Potassium 1329.28mg	38%
Total Carbohydrates 14.83g	5%
Fiber 6.3g	25%
Sugar 6.45g	
Protein 6.91g	14%
MyPoints 1.05	

Recipe Tips

Here is a drink I enjoyed at Hippocrates Institute in south Florida. We serve this twice daily during a detox at our fasting and cleansing center, Detox Oasis.

Green Veggie Juice #2

A refreshing juice without a juicer. As served at DetoxOasis.net.

1-1/2	cup	Kale (or spinach)	6	cups	water
2	ea	apples, medium			

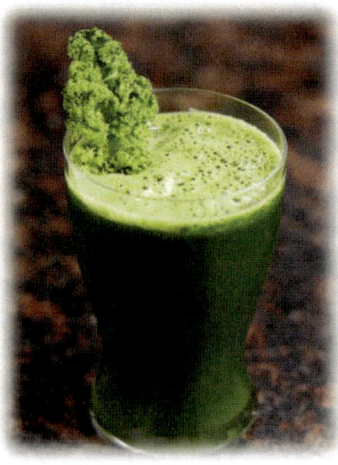

Procedure

1. Blend all ingredients in a Vita-mix or other blender.
2. Pour blended mixture into a nut milk bag.
3. Squeeze mixture over a large bowl and collect the juice.
4. Drink and enjoy!

Equipment Needed:

1. Vita-mix or other strong blender
2. Nut milk bag

Servings: 6

Preparation Time: 5 minutes
Total Time: 5 minutes

Nutrition Facts

Serving size: 1/6 of a recipe (11.1 ounces).

Amount Per Serving	
Calories	39.92
Calories From Fat (4%)	1.76
	% Daily Value
Total Fat 0.22g	<1%
Saturated Fat 0.03g	<1%
Cholesterol 0mg	0%
Sodium 14.92mg	<1%
Potassium 142.16mg	4%
Total Carbohydrates 10.05g	3%
Fiber 1.79g	7%
Sugar 6.3g	
Protein 0.71g	1%
MyPoints 0.46	

Recipe Tips

OK, here is another "Kale Mary, save your life" drink. This drink is so healthy! My only issue with Kale is it does not go through my juicer very well.

High Power Smoothie

As served at FitBodyRetreat.com.

1/2	cup	skim milk*	1	tbsp	protein powder
2/3	cup	plain yogurt, 1%*	1	tsp	agave
2/3	cup	raspberries, frozen (or any berries)	16	oz	water
1	tbsp	flax seeds, ground or whole			

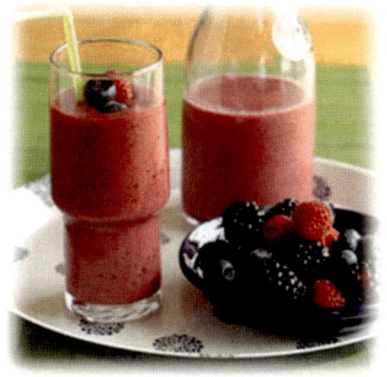

Procedure
1 Blend together all ingredients and serve.

Equipment Needed:
1 Vita-mix or other strong blender

Servings: 1

Preparation Time: 5 minutes
Cooking Time:
Total Time: 5 minutes

Nutrition Facts

Serving size: Entire recipe (39.4 ounces).

Amount Per Serving	
Calories	437.43
Calories From Fat (18%)	76.75
	% Daily Value
Total Fat 8.96g	14%
Saturated Fat 2.15g	11%
Cholesterol 12.25mg	4%
Sodium 336.72mg	14%
Potassium 865.68mg	25%
Total Carbohydrates 72.67g	24%
Fiber 10.61g	42%
Sugar 54.21g	
Protein 22.07g	44%
MyPoints 8.7	

Recipe Tips

Personally, I add a scoop of protein to this smoothie. It's a perfect smoothie following an intense resistance workout. Remember -- after a workout is when you want high protein, high sugar, and low fat for a quick delivery system to your muscles. The rest of the day, you do not need to add the fruit or sugar to the protein as you do not want the calories nor need the quick delivery.

* You can substitute soy versions of these dairy products.

Iced Herbal Coffee

A favorite alternative to a Frappuccino. As served at DetoxOasis.net.

- 1 cup   Teecchino herb coffee, brewed (1/2 tbsp makes 1 cup)
- 3 tsp   almond milk
- 1 tsp   agave (or stevia for less calories)
- 1/2 cup   ice

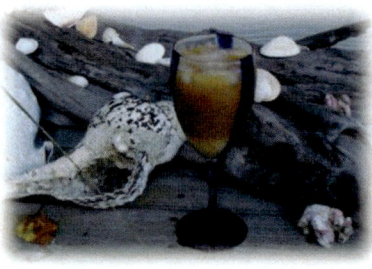

Procedure

1. Blend brewed coffee with other ingredients and serve.

Equipment Needed:

1. Vita-mix or other blender

Servings: 1

Preparation Time: 5 minutes
Cooking Time:
Total Time: 5 minutes

Nutrition Facts

Serving size: Entire recipe (12.3 ounces).

Amount Per Serving	
Calories	31.5
Calories From Fat (0%)	0
	% Daily Value
Total Fat 0g	0%
Sodium 19mg	<1%
Total Carbohydrates 1.5g	<1%
Protein 0g	0%
MyPoints 0.63	

Recipe Tips

I call this the raw foodie coffee. And it's good stuff! Carbs can be your enemy! Beer and bread will never allow you to reach your fat loss goals! I have them on my cheat day only. And if I must use bread for anything, it's only 35-calorie bread that I use.

Real Orange & Fresh

Yummy fresh and sweet! Delicious and fresh! As served at DetoxOasis.net.

1	cup	fresh squeezed orange juice	1/2	cup	ice
5	drops	liquid stevia, vanilla			

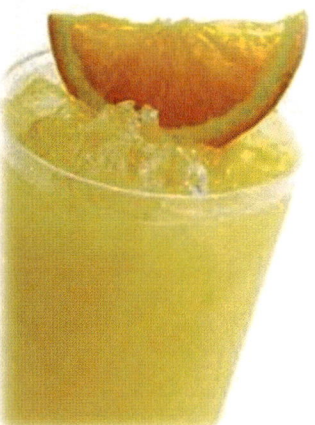

Procedure

1. Peel and juice the oranges.
2. Blend all ingredients using a blender or juicer.

Equipment Needed:

1. Vita-mix or other strong blender, or juicer

Servings: 1

Preparation Time: 5 minutes
Cooking Time:
Total Time: 5 minutes

Nutrition Facts

Serving size: Entire recipe (28.1 ounces).

Amount Per Serving	
Calories	111.6
Calories From Fat (4%)	4.38
	% Daily Value
Total Fat 0.5g	<1%
Saturated Fat 0.06g	<1%
Cholesterol 0mg	0%
Sodium 2.48mg	<1%
Potassium 496mg	14%
Total Carbohydrates 25.79g	9%
Fiber 0.5g	2%
Sugar 20.83g	
Protein 1.74g	3%
MyPoints 2.17	

Seaweed Mineral Drink

A bold RAW drink we serve at the ranch. Loaded with vitamins and minerals. This recipe was brought to us by Kat, a friend and occasionally our raw food chef from Bloomington, Indiana. As served at DetoxOasis.net.

1	ea	apple		1	tbsp	kelp
1	ea	orange		1/2	tsp	garlic
3	ea	dates		1/2	ea	banana
2	tbsp	Spirulina blue green algae powder		1	tbsp	agave
2	tbsp	chlorella				

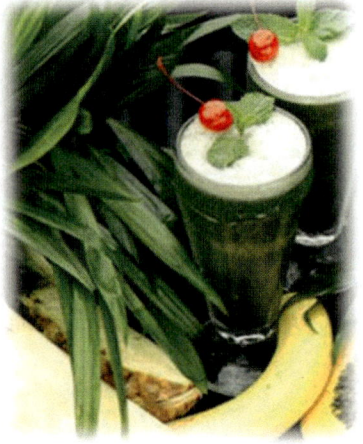

Procedure
1. Place all items in Vita-mix or other blender.
2. Blend well and serve.

Equipment Needed:
1. Vita-mix or other strong blender

Servings: 2

Preparation Time: 5 minutes
Cooking Time:
Total Time: 5 minutes

Nutrition Facts
Serving size: 1/2 of a recipe (20 ounces).

Amount Per Serving	
Calories	239.79
Calories From Fat (2%)	5.44
	% Daily Value
Total Fat 0.56g	<1%
Saturated Fat 0.1g	<1%
Cholesterol 0mg	0%
Sodium 30.59mg	1%
Potassium 445.5mg	13%
Total Carbohydrates 42.94g	14%
Fiber 7.57g	30%
Sugar 20.97g	
Protein 11.38g	23%
MyPoints 4.04	

Recipe Tips
If I was told I only had a few months to live, there are certain foods I would turn to. Just about 100% of them are raw. Raw foods are clean and pure and will heal you, if used correctly. Don't let my occasional negative attitude regarding raw foodists say otherwise. This recipe is one of those, "serious fuel, little fun, high nutrition, save your ass when you are pronounced dying", drinks. Recipe from Kat, friend and client at Spirit Tree Farms in Bloomington, Indiana.

Lunch

Detox Dave

Here are a few things you must consider about muscle with the understanding that muscle burns calories!

Muscle is a metabolically active tissue -- much more so than fat. This means that muscle burns calories even when you're asleep, at rest or at your desk. Simply said, I personally burn more calories than most people at a standing rest. Why? Because I have so much muscle on me. Having more muscle means you can eat more and still lose fat. Muscle is forgiving!

The best way to gain muscle is through resistance training. At the Oasis, we use weights, TRX, Kettle Bells, and P-90X. The methods we use at the Oasis are the same methods you can use at home or at the gym with a personal trainer.

Muscle is what gives your body its shape. You can lose all the fat you want but if you don't have any muscle to show, than you won't have any real shape to show. No real shape is not sexy. Trust me! Here, as you slim up, you really want some lean muscle to give you a long lean shape.

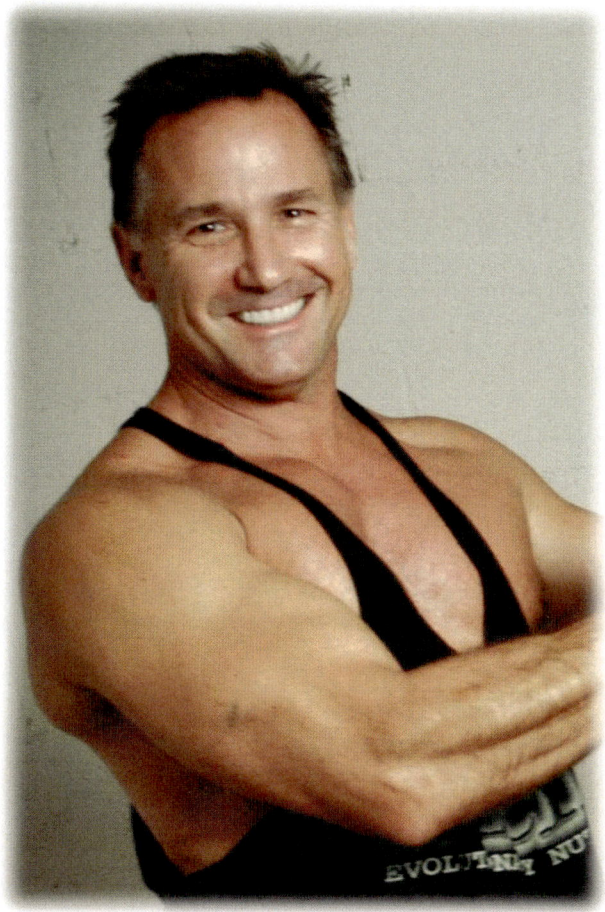

Basil Grilled Chicken

Grilled chicken ready to support your lean muscle needs. As served at FitBodyRetreat.com.

	Non-stick cooking spray	1/2 tsp	basil
4 ea	chicken breasts, skinless, boneless (about 1lb)	1/4 tsp	black pepper

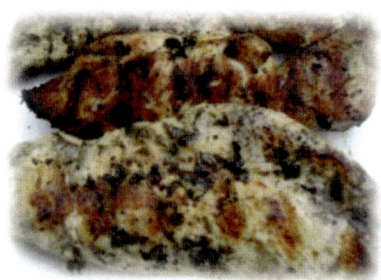

Procedure

1. Heat up your grill to high heat.
2. Spray both sides of your chicken breast.
3. Sprinkle with basil and pepper.
4. Place on grill for 3 min per side.
5. Turn heat to medium and cook an additional 6 min.

Servings: 4

Preparation Time: 5 minutes
Cooking Time: 12 minutes
Total Time: 20 minutes

Nutrition Facts

Serving size: 1/4 of a recipe (7 ounces).

Amount Per Serving	
Calories	284.54
Calories From Fat (21%)	58.4
	% Daily Value
Total Fat 6.15g	9%
Saturated Fat 1.74g	9%
Cholesterol 146.2mg	49%
Sodium 127.44mg	5%
Potassium 446.67mg	13%
Total Carbohydrates 0.17g	<1%
Fiber 0.1g	<1%
Sugar 0g	
Protein 53.41g	107%
MyPoints 6.18	

Recipe Tips

When I cook chicken, I tend to cook 10-12 chicken breasts at a time. From omelets to wraps to a dinner meal or a pure protein snack, I reach for this rather than chips. Plus, it's easier to eat clean if it's already made.

Beef Stew

A nice slow cooker stew that can be made with just about any meat. Juicy and tender! As served at FitBodyRetreat.com.

1	ea	onion
1	lb	roast beef, or beef steak
4	ea	potatoes, cut into 1/2" pieces
1	lb	carrots, cut into 1/2" pieces
2	ea	celery stalks, cut into 1" pieces
1/4	cup	tomato paste
1/2	tsp	black pepper
2	tbsp	Bragg Liquid Aminos
2	tbsp	parsley, finely chopped
4	cups	water

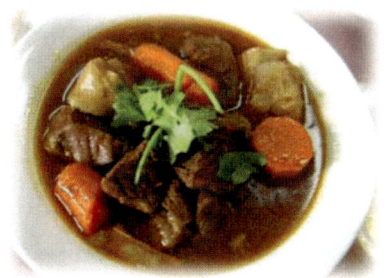

Procedure

1. Place all ingredients in a slow cooker or crockpot.
2. Cook on low for 8-10 hrs. Then serve.

Equipment Needed:

1. Crockpot

Servings: 4

Preparation Time: 20 minutes
Cooking Time: 10 hours
Total Time: 10 hours

Nutrition Facts

Serving size: 1/4 of a recipe (26.3 ounces).

Amount Per Serving	
Calories	454.89
Calories From Fat (30%)	135.88
	% Daily Value
Total Fat 15.66g	24%
Saturated Fat 6.63g	33%
Cholesterol 74.84mg	25%
Sodium 573.38mg	24%
Potassium 1879.87mg	54%
Total Carbohydrates 53.06g	18%
Fiber 9.3g	37%
Sugar 10.67g	
Protein 29.66g	59%
MyPoints 9.6	

Recipe Tips

Remember you can make this with elk, buffalo or the cheapest cut of beef you can find. Cook it a long time on low heat and it will be tasty and tender.

Buffalo Salsa Wrap

A great tasting, high protein wrap. As served at FitBodyRetreat.com.

1/4	lb	buffalo, ground (bison)	1	tbsp	parmesan cheese
1	squirt	Bragg Liquid Aminos	1	tbsp	salsa (30 cal. max)
1/4	cup	spinach	1	ea	tortilla wrap, low calorie
1	ea	tomato, small, cubed			

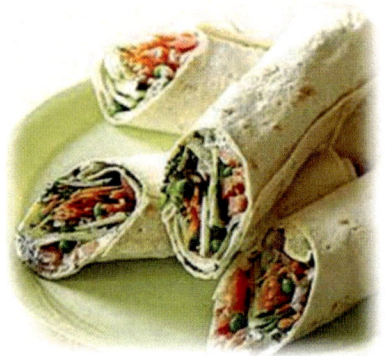

Procedure

1. Form ground buffalo into a patty and grill.
2. After it's cooked, break up the patty.
3. Squirt it with liquid aminos.
4. Add all the ingredients into the wrap.
5. Roll it up, cut and serve.

Servings: 1

Preparation Time: 10 minutes
Cooking Time: 15 minutes
Total Time: 30 minutes

Nutrition Facts

Serving size: Entire recipe (15.3 ounces).

Amount Per Serving	
Calories	156.98
Calories From Fat (46%)	72.99
	% Daily Value
Total Fat 8.67g	13%
Saturated Fat 0.9g	5%
Cholesterol 4.4mg	1%
Sodium 221.92mg	9%
Potassium 311.29mg	9%
Total Carbohydrates 11.02g	4%
Fiber 1.51g	6%
Sugar 2.96g	
Protein 11.43g	23%
MyPoints 3.56	

Recipe Tips

I'm a big fan of wraps. Just make sure you watch the calorie counts on the tortillas – they can vary a lot! Some tortillas can be as high as 300 calories each! Find the low calorie, low carb ones in the refrigerated section at the store. I eat in the same manner for lunch as I do for breakfast. It's not a big event for me. It's only fuel. Lunch is usually 1/2 bag of spinach with Bragg Liquid Aminos, rice vinegar and whatever meat is left over from dinner, or a low carb wrap with the same stuff in it as the salad. Keep it simple and you will stay with your program.

Burrito Protein Power House

Mexican flare with heaps of protein to build that lean muscle! Tortilla, black beans, cottage cheese, quinoa and pico-de-gallo! As served at FitBodyRetreat.com.

4	oz	ground buffalo	1/4	cup	quinoa, cooked*
2	ea	corn tortillas	1/4	cup	black beans, cooked*
1/2	cup	cottage cheese, low fat 1%	1/4	cup	pico-de-gallo*

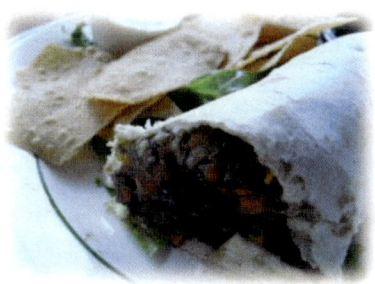

Procedure

1. Place the tortilla on a plate.
2. Add the ground buffalo on the tortilla.
3. Place the quinoa on the tortilla.
4. Pour the black beans on the quinoa.
5. Place a scoop of cottage cheese on the beans.
6. Place the pico-de-gallo on the very top and serve.

Servings: 1

Preparation Time: 10 minutes
Cooking Time: 15 minutes
Total Time: 20 minutes

Nutrition Facts

Serving size: Entire recipe (13.9 ounces).

Amount Per Serving	
Calories	589.06
Calories From Fat (32%)	190.12
	% Daily Value
Total Fat 20.82g	32%
Saturated Fat 0.96g	5%
Cholesterol 4.52mg	2%
Sodium 707.92mg	29%
Potassium 409.46mg	12%
Total Carbohydrates 49.35g	16%
Fiber 7.74g	31%
Sugar 3.07g	
Protein 50.31g	101%
MyPoints 12.72	

Recipe Tips

Take a look at the protein in this dish! Need I say more! DO NOT SKIMP on your protein levels! Protein builds the lean muscle you need to increase your daily calorie burn rate and it makes you feel full.

* See recipe for Quinoa Basic
* See recipe for Black Beans Basic.
* See recipe for Pico-de-Gallo.

Ceviche

A wonderful dish I learned in a shack in Costa Rica. Raw white fish marinated in lime juice with cilantro, onions, tomatoes and red peppers. Great as a snack or an appetizer! As served at FitBodyRetreat.com.

1	ea	cod fillet, small (or other firm fish)	1/2	ea	red pepper
1	handful	shrimp, cooked (about 1 cup)	1	bunch	cilantro, fresh, finely chopped
1	ea	tomato, small	6	ea	limes (juice of 6 limes or more)
1	ea	onion, small	1	cup	ginger ale (optional)

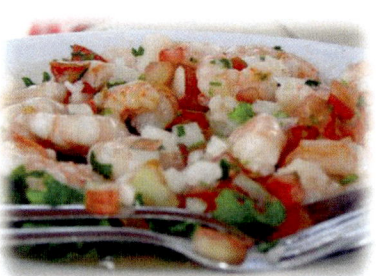

Procedure

1. Cut the fish into 1/2" cubes.
2. De-tail the shrimp.
3. Cut all the veggies into small squares about 1/4 the size of a dime.
4. Chop the cilantro very well.
5. Juice the limes.
6. Add all ingredients together in a bowl or bag, except the ginger ale, and stir or shake well.
7. Place in refrigerator for 4 hrs. The lime juice will "cook" the fish.
8. Stir or shake occasionally during the 4 hrs.
9. Pull from the fridge and add the ginger ale (to limit the tartness).*
10. Stir or shake well.
11. Place back in the refrigerator until ready to eat.
12. Serve with a slotted spoon that allows juice to drain.

Servings: 2

Preparation Time: 10 minutes
Cooking Time: 4 hours
Total Time: 4 hours

Nutrition Facts

Serving size: 1/2 of a recipe (21.2 ounces).

Amount Per Serving	
Calories	309.14
Calories From Fat (8%)	25.99
	% Daily Value
Total Fat 2.98g	5%
Saturated Fat 0.34g	2%
Cholesterol 296.29mg	99%
Sodium 1422.78mg	59%
Potassium 736.35mg	21%
Total Carbohydrates 32.51g	11%
Fiber 2.34g	9%
Sugar 16.85g	
Protein 40.54g	81%
MyPoints 5.96	

Recipe Tips

In a little village on the pacific coast of Costa Rica, while vacationing with good friends, I learned to make this dish. I had not had it before that trip. It's pretty cool how the acid in the lime cooks the fish. Try this dish. Talk about high protein and clean!

* We use the ginger ale to cut the acidic taste of the marinated lime juice and make it less tart.

Chicken & Red Pepper Wrap

As served at FitBodyRetreat.com.

3	oz	skinless, boneless chicken breast, cooked (sliced thinly)
1	tbsp	mayonnaise, light
1	tsp	Dijon mustard
1	ea	tortilla wrap, low calorie
1	ea	lettuce leaf
1/4	cup	quinoa, cooked*
1/4	cup	cucumber
1/4	cup	red pepper

Procedure

1. Mix together mayonnaise and Dijon mustard.
2. Lay tortilla flat, spread evenly with mayonnaise and mustard mixture.
3. Add lettuce leaf on one 1/2 of tortilla.
4. Layer in the quinoa, cucumber, red pepper and chicken on the other 1/2 of tortilla.
5. Fold in the sides and then roll the tortilla.
6. Slice in 1/2 diagonally and serve.

Servings: 1

Preparation Time: 10 minutes
Cooking Time:
Total Time: 10 minutes

Nutrition Facts

Serving size: Entire recipe (7.4 ounces).

Amount Per Serving	
Calories	241.93
Calories From Fat (39%)	93.96
	% Daily Value
Total Fat 10.49g	16%
Saturated Fat 1.61g	8%
Cholesterol 77.54mg	26%
Sodium 185.29mg	8%
Potassium 244.93mg	7%
Total Carbohydrates 7.56g	3%
Fiber 0.15g	<1%
Sugar 0.71g	
Protein 29.61g	59%
MyPoints 5.68	

Recipe Tips

If you enter everything you eat into a foods computer tracking program such as FitDay.com every day for two weeks (14 days), you will realize a simple fact -- you are a creature of habit -- a creature that eats the same foods over and over again -- both good foods and bad. After you determine what it is that you eat on a regular basis, it becomes easy to make small adjustments. Now you may dial in your calories, fats, and protein numbers, exactly where they belong for you. Treat your body as you would a sales or financial report, and you will automatically start to trend to better numbers. When you are aware of a trend, it's easier to fix the trend. What is the first thing you do at work when you want to understand what's going on? -- You look at the numbers.

* See recipe for Quinoa Basic.

Chicken Caesar Wrap

A basic low carbohydrate/low calorie wrap! As served at FitBodyRetreat.com.

4	oz	chicken breast, cooked, diced	1	squirt	Bragg Liquid Aminos
1	cup	spinach	1	tbsp	Caesar dressing, low calorie (25 cal. max)
1/4	ea	red pepper	1	ea	tortilla wrap, low calorie, low carb
1	ea	green onion			
1/4	cup	alfalfa sprouts (or sunflower)			

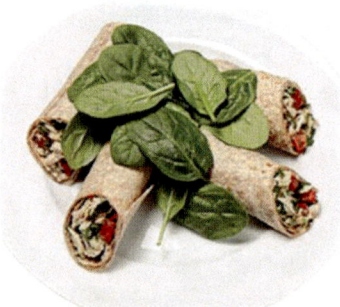

Procedure

1. Place all the ingredients in the wrap.
2. Squirt liquid aminos over the ingredients.
3. Add the Caesar dressing, and serve.

Servings: 1

Preparation Time: 5 minutes
Cooking Time:
Total Time: 10 minutes

Nutrition Facts

Serving size: Entire recipe (18.4 ounces).

Amount Per Serving	
Calories	278.26
Calories From Fat (25%)	68.64
	% Daily Value
Total Fat 7.8g	12%
Saturated Fat 1.18g	6%
Cholesterol 96.39mg	32%
Sodium 148.07mg	6%
Potassium 577.38mg	16%
Total Carbohydrates 13.67g	5%
Fiber 1.83g	7%
Sugar 2.01g	
Protein 39.93g	80%
MyPoints 5.85	

Recipe Tips

Remember -- you can use whatever leftover meat you have in the fridge. Just don't use packaged meat. Also, don't mess it up with bad condiments! That's where most people fail. This is quite possibly my favorite wrap. Why? Because I have so much chicken in my fridge cooked up in advance, I have to use it up in every dish I can until it's all gone!

Chicken Tofu Pizza

As served at FitBodyRetreat.com.

1	ea	pizza crust, whole wheat		1	oz	mozzarella cheese, skim
3	tbsp	tomato sauce, no sugar added		1/2	tsp	macadamia nut oil
2	oz	tofu, firm, sliced		1/2	cup	red pepper, sliced
2	oz	chicken, breast, cooked		1/2	cup	fresh spinach leaves, trimmed and torn

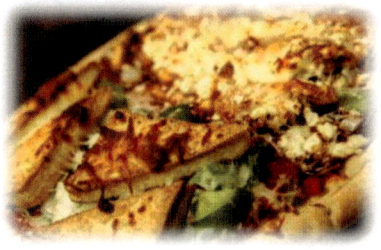

Procedure

1. Heat oil in a pan and sauté the vegetables lightly.
2. Spread the tomato sauce over the pizza crust.
3. Place ingredients on pizza and top with cheese.
4. Bake in oven at 375F until done, about 8-12 minutes.

Servings: 1

Oven Temperature: 375°F

Preparation Time: 10 minutes
Cooking Time: 15 minutes
Total Time: 30 minutes

Nutrition Facts

Serving size: Entire recipe (12.4 ounces).

Amount Per Serving	
Calories	645.89
Calories From Fat (28%)	177.72
	% Daily Value
Total Fat 20.46g	31%
Saturated Fat 3.78g	19%
Cholesterol 66.34mg	22%
Sodium 1176.38mg	49%
Potassium 576.62mg	16%
Total Carbohydrates 73.71g	25%
Fiber 2.21g	9%
Sugar 4.55g	
Protein 47.56g	95%
MyPoints 14.18	

Recipe Tips

One of my Detox Oasis interns showed me this dish. It's very good!

Elk & Lentil Burritos

We're continually trying to incorporate healthy, tasty meals into our menus. Both kids and adults love these mildly spiced burritos that combine filling lentils with crisp zucchini. As served at FitBodyRetreat.com.

2	cups	water	1	cup	taco sauce
1	cup	dried lentils	1	cup	mozzarella cheese, part skim, shredded
2	tbsp	dried minced onion	1	lb	ground buffalo, cooked (or elk which is leaner)
1/2	tsp	dried minced garlic			
1/2	tsp	ground cumin	8	ea	tortilla wrap, low calorie
1/8	tsp	hot pepper sauce			
1	ea	zucchini, small, chopped			

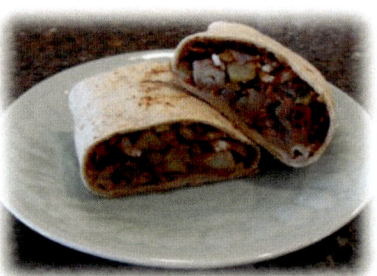

Procedure

1. In a saucepan, combine the first 6 ingredients and bring to a boil.
2. Reduce heat, cover and simmer for 15-20 min or until lentils are tender.
3. Drain if necessary.
4. Stir in zucchini, taco sauce and cheese.
5. Add cooked ground buffalo (or elk).
6. Place about 1/2 cupfuls of the mixture down the center of each tortilla.
7. Fold sides and ends over filling, roll up and serve.

Servings: 8

Preparation Time: 10 minutes
Cooking Time: 15 minutes
Total Time: 25 minutes

Nutrition Facts

Serving size: 1/8 of a recipe (11 ounces).

Amount Per Serving	
Calories	332.6
Calories From Fat (38%)	125.84
	% Daily Value
Total Fat 14.22g	22%
Saturated Fat 1.72g	9%
Cholesterol 10.56mg	4%
Sodium 359.96mg	15%
Potassium 304.88mg	9%
Total Carbohydrates 25.13g	8%
Fiber 7.76g	31%
Sugar 3.49g	
Protein 27.44g	55%
MyPoints 7.04	

Recipe Tips

If you are eating this dish, then you know your protein and are into eating the tastiest red meat on the planet! Quick note for protein junkies -- not all protein shakes and bars are created equal! Look at calories and protein counts before you consume anything! Some flavors from the same manufacturer of shakes and bars will have different calories. When you switch from chocolate to vanilla, make sure you read the label's nutritional counts.

Elk Chili

A simple but tasty chili recipe using ground elk meat as the base. Best served with a low calorie spinach salad. As served at FitBodyRetreat.com.

2-1/2	lbs	ground elk	1-1/2	tbsp	chili powder
2	ea	yellow onions, large, diced	1-1/2	tsp	ground cumin
6	ea	tomatoes, large, diced	1	tbsp	Bragg Liquid Aminos
2	ea	red peppers, large	1	tsp	black pepper
16	oz	black beans, fresh (soaked overnight and drained)	1	tsp	dried oregano
1	ea	hot pepper, seeds removed and diced small	1/4	cup	agave

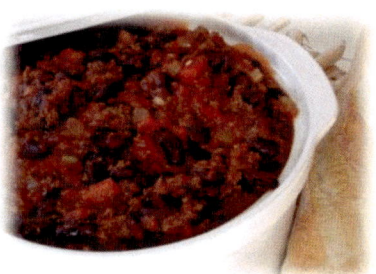

Procedure

1. In a large deep skillet over medium heat, cook the ground elk with the diced onions until evenly browned.
2. Drain off excess grease.
3. Pour the tomatoes, red peppers, black beans and hot pepper into the skillet with the meat.
4. Stir to blend.
5. Season with chili powder, cumin, liquid aminos, pepper, oregano, and agave.
6. Cover and simmer over low heat for at least 1-1/2 hr.

Servings: 10

Preparation Time: 30 minutes
Cooking Time: 1 hour
Total Time: 2 hours

Nutrition Facts

Serving size: 1/10 of a recipe (16.1 ounces).

Amount Per Serving	
Calories	292.8
Calories From Fat (12%)	36.44
	% Daily Value
Total Fat 3.78g	6%
Saturated Fat 1.38g	7%
Cholesterol 79.38mg	26%
Sodium 235.98mg	10%
Potassium 840.86mg	24%
Total Carbohydrates 21.06g	7%
Fiber 3.08g	12%
Sugar 5.61g	
Protein 38.77g	78%
MyPoints 5.56	

Recipe Tips

Perfect for a winter day and perfect fuel for building lean muscle! Brad Simms, our Elk Ridge executive chef at one time, taught us this dish.

Elk Garlic BBQ Burger

Grass-fed, organic elk! As served at FitBodyRetreat.com.

6	oz	elk, ground	1/2	ea	tomato, small, sliced
1	tsp	garlic, chopped	1/4	cup	alfalfa sprouts
2	slices	bread, low calorie (35 cal. max)	1	tbsp	mustard*
1	tsp	BBQ sauce (Sweet Baby Ray's, 16 cal. max)	1	squirt	Bragg Liquid Aminos

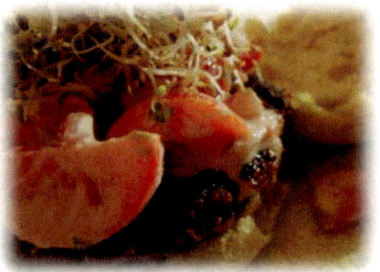

Procedure

1. Mix the garlic into the ground elk as you form it into a patty.
2. Grill the burger.
3. Place burger on bread.
4. Spread on the BBQ sauce.
5. Add vegetables, liquid aminos, and serve.

Servings: 1

Preparation Time: 10 minutes
Cooking Time: 15 minutes
Total Time: 30 minutes

Nutrition Facts

Serving size: Entire recipe (15.7 ounces).

Amount Per Serving	
Calories	349.97
Calories From Fat (14%)	48.09
	% Daily Value
Total Fat 5.55g	9%
Saturated Fat 2g	10%
Cholesterol 119.07mg	40%
Sodium 543.9mg	23%
Potassium 791.83mg	23%
Total Carbohydrates 22.7g	8%
Fiber 1.28g	5%
Sugar 1.37g	
Protein 55.69g	111%
MyPoints 7.21	

Recipe Tips

Add BBQ sauce to a pinecone, and it would no doubt taste good. Be careful on condiments. Most of us use way too much. Measure out the BBQ sauce. You will be surprised how much flavor you can get out of a teaspoon full!

* Use mustard or other low calorie condiments. Stay away from high fat, high calorie condiments!

Fish Cakes

Delicious appetizer! As served at FitBodyRetreat.com.

2	handfuls	cod (or any white fish - about 2 cups)	2	tbsp	fish sauce
2	tbsp	red curry paste	1	tbsp	agave
4	ea	kaffir lime leaves*	2	tbsp	macadamia nut oil (use for frying method)
1/2	handful	snow peas (or green beans - about 1/4 cup)			

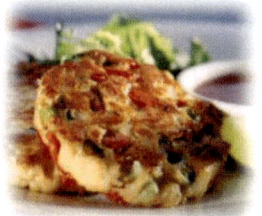

Procedure

1. Add fish to a Vita-mix or other blender and blend.
2. Add red curry paste and mix again.
3. Transfer fish from blender to large bowl.
4. Add remaining ingredients to bowl and mix well.
5. Form into balls.
6. Press to form patties that are 1/2" thick and 2" round.
7. Fry in oil until done or spray a baking sheet with non-stick spray and bake at 425F for 8-12 min.

Equipment Needed:

1. Vita-mix or other strong blender

Servings: 2

Oven Temperature: 425°F

Preparation Time: 10 minutes
Cooking Time: 12 minutes
Total Time: 30 minutes

Nutrition Facts

Serving size: 1/2 of a recipe (22.4 ounces).

Amount Per Serving	
Calories	271.85
Calories From Fat (56%)	151.58
	% Daily Value
Total Fat 14.86g	23%
Saturated Fat 0.17g	<1%
Cholesterol 54.83mg	18%
Sodium 1765.78mg	74%
Potassium 578.42mg	17%
Total Carbohydrates 2.91g	<1%
Fiber 0g	0%
Sugar 0.66g	
Protein 23.62g	47%
MyPoints 6.68	

Recipe Tips

Saturday night is a great night to cheat with your diet! Once a week is ok. For people with weekends off, Saturday is the day where all seems normal in your food world. It's ok to have pizza and beer! When you cheat, do it right! Fish cakes don't count for a good cheat! You want high fat high carb foods for a really good cheat!

* Kaffir lime leaves are practically impossible to find in the USA. We grow our own Kaffir lime tree indoors here at the ranch. You can substitute 1 fresh kaffir lime leaf with several dried. If you can't find the leaves at all, you may substitute with regular lime zest or juice, but I guarantee that you will never be able to replace exactly the perfumy note that the kaffir leaf is recognized for. Once you have found fresh leaves, freeze some for later. They will last for several months in the freezer. In fact, you can sometimes find them already frozen in the stores.

Lettuce Tofu Veggie Wraps

As served at FitBodyRetreat.com.

2	ea	lettuce leaves, medium
1/2	cup	tofu, firm, diced
1/3	cup	broccoli, diced
1/3	cup	red pepper, diced
1/3	cup	alfalfa sprouts (or sunflower)
1	tbsp	apple cider vinegar
1	tbsp	Bragg Liquid Aminos
1	ea	pear, whole

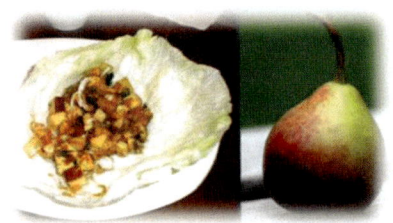

Procedure

1. Place tofu and veggies on lettuce leaves.
2. Mix apple cider vinegar and liquid aminos together for dressing.
3. Drizzle dressing on top.
4. Wrap up like a burrito and serve with pear on the side.

Servings: 1

Preparation Time: 10 minutes
Cooking Time:
Total Time: 10 minutes

Nutrition Facts

Serving size: Entire recipe (15.1 ounces).

Amount Per Serving	
Calories	231.34
Calories From Fat (24%)	55.24
	% Daily Value
Total Fat 7.03g	11%
Saturated Fat 0.65g	3%
Cholesterol 0mg	0%
Sodium 505.5mg	21%
Potassium 552.67mg	16%
Total Carbohydrates 33.92g	11%
Fiber 6.87g	27%
Sugar 19.51g	
Protein 16.5g	33%
MyPoints 4.41	

Recipe Tips

These are fun to make and are not filling. Impress your vegan friends with this dish.

Lettuce Veggie Wraps

Raw veggies inside of lettuce wrapped up like a taco. As served at DetoxOasis.net.

2	ea	avocados, ripe	1/4	cup	fresh cilantro, chopped
3	ea	tomatoes, diced	1	ea	kernels from a fresh ear of corn
1/2	ea	jalapeno pepper, diced			
2	tbsp	yellow onion, diced	2	tsp	fresh lime juice
3	ea	garlic cloves, minced	6-8	ea	lettuce leaves

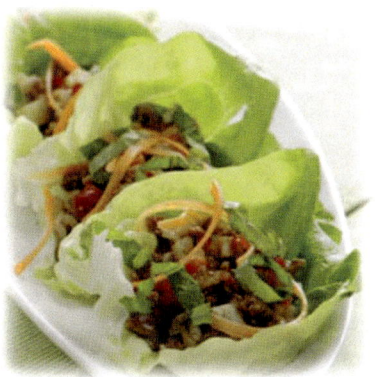

Procedure

1. In a medium sized bowl, mash the avocado.
2. Add remaining ingredients and stir until well mixed.
3. Spread 2-3 tbsp of this mixture onto lettuce leaves and wrap.

Servings: 2

Preparation Time: 20 minutes
Cooking Time:
Total Time: 20 minutes

Nutrition Facts

Serving size: 1/2 of a recipe (18.7 ounces).

Amount Per Serving	
Calories	438.97
Calories From Fat (56%)	247.75
	% Daily Value
Total Fat 30.49g	47%
Saturated Fat 4.42g	22%
Cholesterol 0mg	0%
Sodium 41.61mg	2%
Potassium 1783.52mg	51%
Total Carbohydrates 44.05g	15%
Fiber 18.65g	75%
Sugar 9.99g	
Protein 8.9g	18%
MyPoints 10.52	

Quinoa, Beans & Elk

High protein combo to pack on that muscle! As served at FitBodyRetreat.com.

2 oz	elk burger, cooked*	
1/4 cup	quinoa, cooked*	
1/4 cup	black beans, fresh, cooked*	
2 tbsp	pico-de-gallo*	

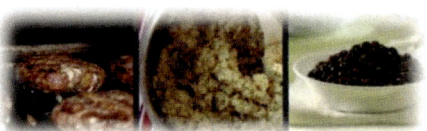

Procedure

1. After everything is cooked, place elk burger on bed of quinoa.
2. Top with black beans and pico-de-gallo.

Servings: 1

Preparation Time: 5 minutes
Cooking Time:
Total Time: 5 minutes

Nutrition Facts

Serving size: Entire recipe (12.1 ounces).

Amount Per Serving	
Calories	299.24
Calories From Fat (13%)	39.05
	% Daily Value
Total Fat 4.4g	7%
Saturated Fat 1.01g	5%
Cholesterol 39.69mg	13%
Sodium 114.31mg	5%
Potassium 606.82mg	17%
Total Carbohydrates 39.46g	13%
Fiber 6.72g	27%
Sugar 0g	
Protein 26.51g	53%
MyPoints 5.55	

Recipe Tips

Now here is a high protein packed meal. You will love it!

* See recipe for Turkey-Elk-Buffalo-Beef Burger Grilled.
* See recipe for Quinoa Basic.
* See recipe for Black Beans Basic.
* See recipe for Pico-de-Gallo.

Raw-Fajita Alternative

A great alternative to the standard fajita. As service at DetoxOasis.net.

- 2 ea portabella mushroom caps
- 1 ea red onion, medium
- 1 ea red pepper
- 1 ea yellow bell pepper
- 3/4 cup extra virgin olive oil
- 1/3 cup Bragg Liquid Aminos
- 1/4 cup cumin
- 4 ea lettuce leaves, large (or Collard, Romaine, etc.)

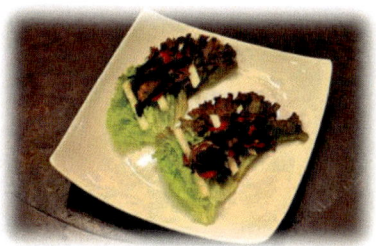

Procedure

1. Slice peppers, mushrooms and onion into long thin strips.
2. Mix all ingredients in a bowl except for lettuce leaves.
3. Pour mixture into a zip lock bag.
4. Refrigerate this marinated mix for 6 hrs, turning bag often.
5. Serve the marinated mix in the lettuce leaves. Wrap up like a fajita.

Servings: 4

Preparation Time: 20 minutes
Cooking Time: 6 hours
Total Time: 6 hours and 30 minutes

Nutrition Facts

Serving size: 1/4 of a recipe (9.2 ounces).

Amount Per Serving	
Calories	431.2
Calories From Fat (82%)	353.85
	% Daily Value
Total Fat 42.37g	65%
Saturated Fat 5.76g	29%
Cholesterol 0mg	0%
Sodium 664.17mg	28%
Potassium 573.15mg	16%
Total Carbohydrates 12.9g	4%
Fiber 3.38g	14%
Sugar 3.75g	
Protein 7.94g	16%
MyPoints 11.48	

Recipe Tips

There are really good. What makes or breaks this dish is the onion. Try and go with a sweet Vidalia onion. If the onion is too hot, it overpowers the dish and then it's just too much onion flavor.

Raw-Garden Burgers

This recipe brings the garden to the burger! As served at DetoxOasis.net.

6	tbsp	water	1	cup	shelled sunflower seeds, ground	
3	tbsp	flax seeds, ground				
1	handful	parsley, fresh (or 4 tbsp fresh or 4 tsp dried)	1/2	cup	celery, finely chopped	
			6	tbsp	green onion, chopped	
			2	tbsp	red pepper, chopped	
1	cup	carrot pulp*	2	tsp	Bragg Liquid Aminos	

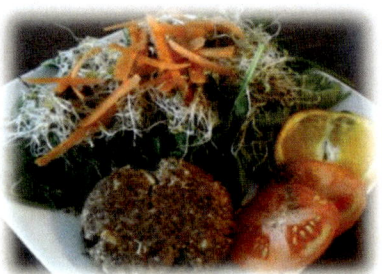

Procedure

1. Grind flax seeds in a coffee grinder.
2. In your Vita-mix or blender - combine the water and the ground flax seeds and blend well.
3. Pour mixture into a bowl - set aside.
4. In a separate bowl - mix carrot pulp, sunflower seeds, parsley, celery, onion, pepper and liquid aminos.
5. Add flax seed mixture to other ingredients.
6. Form into 6 patties about 1/2" thick. (if you need more water, add enough to make a good patty)
7. Dehydrate at 110 degrees for 4-8 hours.

Equipment Needed:

1. Coffee grinder
2. Vita-mix or other strong blender
3. Dehydrator

Servings: 6

Preparation Time: 30 minutes
Cooking Time: 8 hours
Total Time: 8 hours

Nutrition Facts

Serving size: 1/6 of a recipe (2.5 ounces).

Amount Per Serving	
Calories	89.8
Calories From Fat (61%)	54.45
	% Daily Value
Total Fat 6.58g	10%
Saturated Fat 0.58g	3%
Cholesterol 0mg	0%
Sodium 79.46mg	3%
Potassium 220.86mg	6%
Total Carbohydrates 6.13g	2%
Fiber 3.28g	13%
Sugar 1.64g	
Protein 3.48g	7%
MyPoints 1.69	

Recipe Tips

Veggie burgers are a great alternative to meat. Just make sure you drink a protein shake with it to maintain your desired protein levels.

* To make carrot pulp - juice some carrots and use the pulp that is remaining.

Raw-Zucchini Pasta

A simple pasta alternative with our Spaghetti Sauce or Raw Alfredo Sauce. As served at DetoxOasis.net.

1 ea zucchini, raw

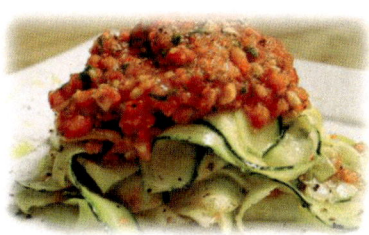

Procedure

1. Peel the skin off the zucchini with a vegetable peeler.
2. Peel the zucchini down to the seeds.
3. Place the peelings in a bowl.
4. Serve with our Spaghetti Sauce or Raw Alfredo Sauce.

Servings: 1

Preparation Time: 5 minutes
Cooking Time: 5 minutes
Total Time: 5 minutes

Nutrition Facts

Serving size: Entire recipe (6.9 ounces).

Amount Per Serving	
Calories	33.32
Calories From Fat (16%)	5.33
	% Daily Value
Total Fat 0.63g	<1%
Saturated Fat 0.16g	<1%
Cholesterol 0mg	0%
Sodium 15.68mg	<1%
Potassium 511.56mg	15%
Total Carbohydrates 6.1g	2%
Fiber 1.96g	8%
Sugar 4.9g	
Protein 2.37g	5%
MyPoints 0.33	

Recipe Tips

I love raw foods! But I also eat a balance of cooked foods. My rule of thumb is this: when I meet someone who looks amazing, I like to ask them about their diet. It is the person that looks amazing that you will learn the most from regarding how you too may improve your diet and your look! Take a look at the raw foodie Jenna Norwood down Sarasota way. She's quite possibly one of the fittest and sexiest raw ladies out there. She has some amazing videos and books published. Check out her work. Kelly Serbonich, former chef at Hippocrates Institute in South Florida, first introduced me to raw pasta here at my ranch in Indiana. Together, we did a short local television show on raw foods.

Red Pepper Stuffed & Chicken Salad

As served at FitBodyRetreat.com.

1	ea	red pepper, large	1/3	cup	cucumber, diced
3	oz	chicken, cooked, diced	1	tbsp	mayonnaise, light
1/2	cup	celery, diced	1/4	tsp	black pepper
6	ea	black olives			

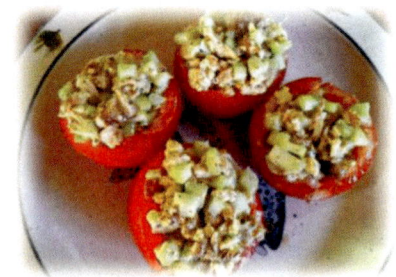

Procedure

1. Slice the red pepper in half, remove seeds.
2. Combine the remaining ingredients and mix well.
3. Fill the two red pepper halves with the mixture.

Servings: 1

Preparation Time: 10 minutes
Cooking Time:
Total Time: 10 minutes

Nutrition Facts

Serving size: Entire recipe (13.3 ounces).

Amount Per Serving	
Calories	282.01
Calories From Fat (37%)	104.32
	% Daily Value
Total Fat 11.36g	17%
Saturated Fat 2.05g	10%
Cholesterol 77.54mg	26%
Sodium 467.44mg	19%
Potassium 757.05mg	22%
Total Carbohydrates 14.72g	5%
Fiber 5.31g	21%
Sugar 8.44g	
Protein 28.82g	58%
MyPoints 5.79	

Recipe Tips

I grew up on my mom's hamburger stuffed green bell peppers. This one blows away mom's old recipe.

Turkey Sandwich

A quick sandwich that tastes great! As served at FitBodyRetreat.com.

4	oz	turkey, cooked*	1	tbsp	mustard*
1	ea	tomato, small	1/4	cup	carrots, shredded
1/2	cup	alfalfa sprouts	2	slices	bread, low calorie (35 cal. max)

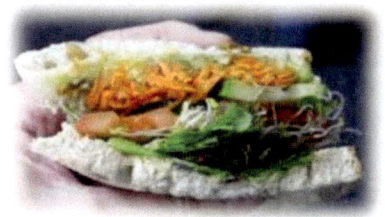

Procedure

1 Layer the ingredients into a sandwich and enjoy!

Servings: 1

Preparation Time: 5 minutes
Cooking Time:
Total Time: 5 minutes

Nutrition Facts

Serving size: Entire recipe (9.5 ounces).

Amount Per Serving	
Calories	304.7
Calories From Fat (19%)	58.26
	% Daily Value
Total Fat 6.62g	10%
Saturated Fat 1.74g	9%
Cholesterol 86.18mg	29%
Sodium 481.3mg	20%
Potassium 676.21mg	19%
Total Carbohydrates 23.35g	8%
Fiber 2.69g	11%
Sugar 3.86g	
Protein 39.65g	79%
MyPoints 6.11	

Recipe Tips

This is a standard healthy sandwich. You can alter your meat and toppings as long as they are not processed. It's the bread that will crush any weight loss or fat loss program. I use 35/40 calorie bread for my sandwiches.

* Do not use packaged turkey as sodium is too high.
* Most people destroy the calorie content of this sandwich with the wrong condiment. If mustard will not work for you, find something that will. Mayonnaise is out of the question. Try Bragg Liquid Aminos. It's hard to beat 0 calories.

Turkey Sandwich - Multigrain

As served at FitBodyRetreat.com.

3	oz	turkey breast, roasted, sliced*	1	bunch	spinach (or mixed greens, about 1 cup)
2	slices	bread, multigrain	1	tbsp	cream cheese, light
1/3	ea	tomato, medium, sliced thinly	1	tbsp	Dijon mustard

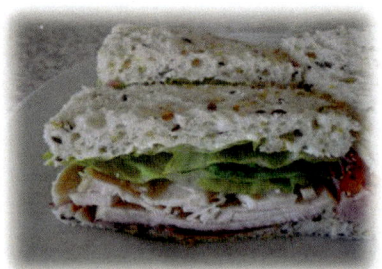

Procedure

1. Spread cream cheese on one slice of bread and mustard on the other.
2. Layer the ingredients evenly and serve.

Servings: 1

Preparation Time: 5 minutes
Cooking Time:
Total Time: 5 minutes

Nutrition Facts

Serving size: Entire recipe (13.6 ounces).

Amount Per Serving	
Calories	330.89
Calories From Fat (21%)	67.86
	% Daily Value
Total Fat 8.12g	12%
Saturated Fat 1.43g	7%
Cholesterol 8.1mg	3%
Sodium 638.65mg	27%
Potassium 323.09mg	9%
Total Carbohydrates 34.73g	12%
Fiber 1.67g	7%
Sugar 2.21g	
Protein 36.08g	72%
MyPoints 6.96	

Recipe Tips

My son, Rob, prefers the multigrain bread. He won't touch the 35-calorie bread unless it's all we have. At age 17, he was 5'9", weighed 180 pounds and could bench press 305 pounds. He eats clean and presently doesn't need to worry too much about his bread or carbs. His protein daily intake is 250 grams as his goal is to pack on a lot of muscle.

* Do not use packaged turkey as the sodium is too high.

Turkey-Elk-Buffalo-Beef Burger Grilled

Regardless of what type of meat you use for your burger, season all the same. Just be careful of the time with the more gamey meats and it will turn out fine! As served at FitBodyRetreat.com.

| 1 | lb | ground buffalo*, elk, turkey or beef |
| 1 | dash | black pepper |

Non-stick cooking spray

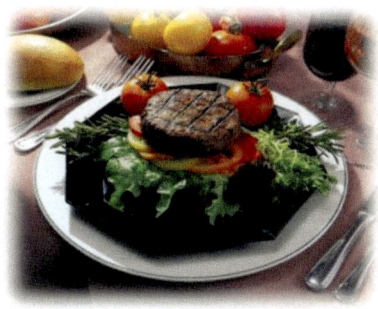

Procedure

1. Form meat into hamburger patties.
2. Season with pepper.
3. Heat grill to high.
4. Sear each side for 2 min.
5. Turn heat to medium and cook for another 6 min.

Servings: 4

Preparation Time: 5 minutes
Cooking Time: 10 minutes
Total Time: 15 minutes

Nutrition Facts

Serving size: 1/4 of a recipe (4.9 ounces).

Amount Per Serving	
Calories	63.06
Calories From Fat (66%)	41.47
	% Daily Value
Total Fat 4.5g	7%
Saturated Fat 0g	0%
Cholesterol 0mg	0%
Sodium 19mg	<1%
Potassium 0.33mg	<1%
Total Carbohydrates 0.02g	<1%
Fiber 0.01g	<1%
Sugar 0g	
Protein 5.25g	11%
MyPoints 1.63	

Recipe Tips

Remember, just because it's a burger doesn't mean you need the bun! If my wife gets stuck in a situation where she must go to McDonald's, she will order a plain chicken sandwich and throw away the bun. It's the protein that makes you full and feel satisfied. It's the bread or bun that will make you crave more carbs.

* Buffalo and elk should never be cooked past medium rare as they are extremely lean and ten to toughen up pretty quickly. Adjust the cooking times as needed to have the best cooked burger.

White Chili - Turkey

As served at FitBodyRetreat.com.

1	tbsp	macadamia nut oil	1/2	tsp	chili powder
16	oz	ground turkey breast	1/4	tsp	cayenne pepper
1	ea	white onion, minced	1	tsp	wine vinegar
2	ea	garlic clove, minced	1/2	tsp	coriander
16	oz	kidney beans, fresh cooked, drained	1/2	tsp	turmeric
28	oz	crushed tomatoes, fresh	1	tbsp	Bragg Liquid Aminos
1/2	cup	chick peas, fresh	5	tbsp	cheddar cheese, shredded, reduced fat

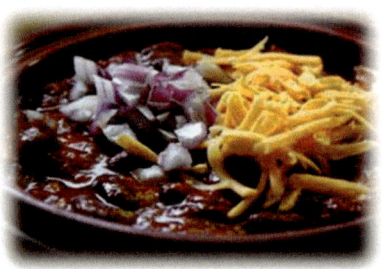

Procedure

1. Heat oil in a large saucepan.
2. Add turkey, onion and garlic.
3. Cook for 5-7 minutes, stirring often.
4. Stir in remaining ingredients, except cheese.
5. Simmer uncovered for 25 minutes.
6. Serve in bowls and top with 1 tbsp of grated cheddar cheese.

Servings: 5

Preparation Time: 10 minutes
Cooking Time: 20 minutes
Total Time: 30 minutes

Nutrition Facts

Serving size: 1/5 of a recipe (14.2 ounces).

Amount Per Serving	
Calories	426.18
Calories From Fat (25%)	108.61
	% Daily Value
Total Fat 12.61g	19%
Saturated Fat 2.49g	12%
Cholesterol 64.66mg	22%
Sodium 420.51mg	18%
Potassium 1284.98mg	37%
Total Carbohydrates 47.66g	16%
Fiber 12.98g	52%
Sugar 3.56g	
Protein 35.3g	71%
MyPoints 8.77	

Recipe Tips

My old friend, Kevin Dorr, who now lives in Denver, first served me this dish in Brighton, Michigan one cold winter evening. This yummy dish will warm you up and is a great alternative to your mom's old recipe. It just may be his evil ex-wife's recipe but don't tell her!

Dinner

Grass Fed Meat

Our objective with the food we serve is to please the client at our center. Daily we serve them perfect meals loaded with serious fat burning and muscle building fuel.

Each day at the Oasis, we try to choose foods that will propel our clients towards their health and fitness goals faster than they could have imagined. And along that path, to teach them how to add more lean muscle both during their stay at our center and back at home.

We teach our clients and staff how to prepare all the foods in the book for lifelong skill sets.

The foods that we prepare are based on target that I try to maintain as close to what the experts refer to as a perfect blend of proteins, carbohydrates and fats.

Our goal at the Oasis is to get as close to a perfect 40/40/20 breakdown in all of our meals.

This means our foods are prepared with a goal of:

- 40% lean protein
- 40% low glycemic carbohydrates
- 20% healthy or good fats

Note the word "goal". At the Oasis, we can hit that goal perfect every time. Once you're at home, do what you can to hit this goal. If your meals are not a perfect balance right away, strive to improve the balance. If you wait for your foods to be perfect, you may never get started. Start cleaning up your diet today. You will perfect it as time passes!

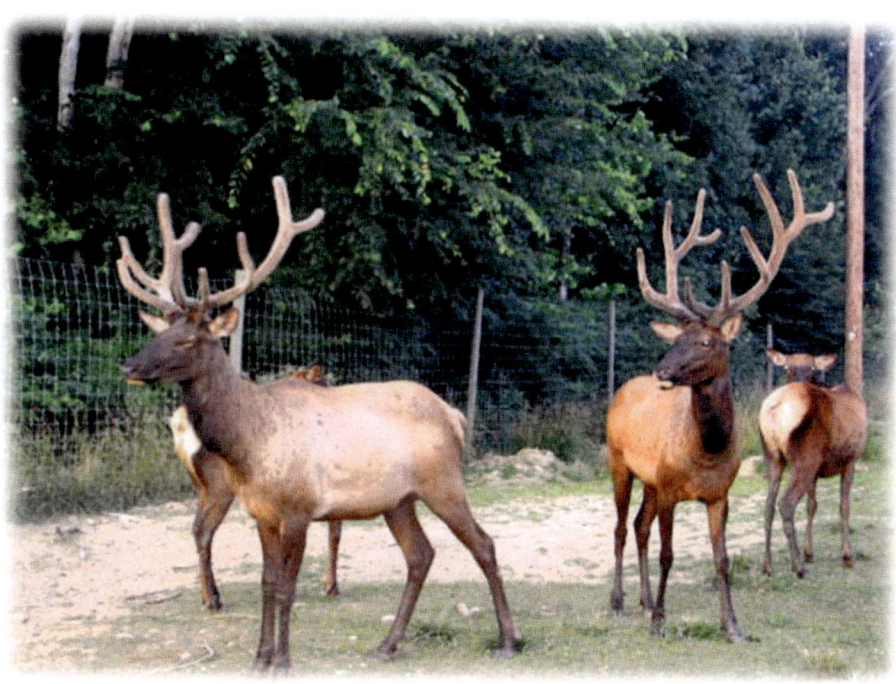

Basil Grilled Chicken

Grilled chicken ready to support your lean muscle needs. As served at FitBodyRetreat.com.

	Non-stick cooking spray	1/2 tsp	basil
4 ea	chicken breasts, skinless, boneless (about 1lb)	1/4 tsp	black pepper

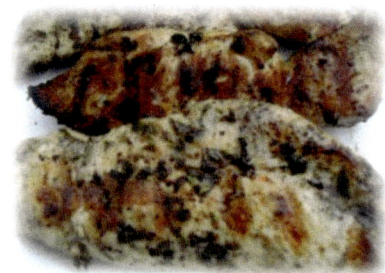

Procedure

1. Heat up your grill to high heat.
2. Spray both sides of your chicken breast.
3. Sprinkle with basil and pepper.
4. Place on grill for 3 min per side.
5. Turn heat to medium and cook an additional 6 min.

Servings: 4

Preparation Time: 5 minutes
Cooking Time: 12 minutes
Total Time: 20 minutes

Nutrition Facts

Serving size: 1/4 of a recipe (7 ounces).

Amount Per Serving	
Calories	284.54
Calories From Fat (21%)	58.4
	% Daily Value
Total Fat 6.15g	9%
Saturated Fat 1.74g	9%
Cholesterol 146.2mg	49%
Sodium 127.44mg	5%
Potassium 446.67mg	13%
Total Carbohydrates 0.17g	<1%
Fiber 0.1g	<1%
Sugar 0g	
Protein 53.41g	107%
MyPoints 6.18	

Recipe Tips

When I cook up chicken, I tend to cook 10-12 chicken breasts at a time. From omelets to wraps to a dinner meal or a pure protein snack, I reach for this rather than chips. Plus, it's easier to eat clean if it's already made.

Beef Stew

A nice slow cooker stew that can be made with just about any meat. Juicy and tender! As served at FitBodyRetreat.com.

1	ea	onion
1	lb	roast beef, or beef steak
4	ea	potatoes, cut into 1/2" pieces
1	lb	carrots, cut into 1/2" pieces
2	ea	celery stalks, cut into 1" pieces
1/4	cup	tomato paste
1/2	tsp	black pepper
2	tbsp	Bragg Liquid Aminos
2	tbsp	parsley, finely chopped
4	cups	water

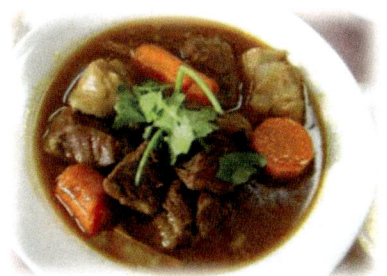

Procedure

1. Place all ingredients in a slow cooker or crockpot.
2. Cook on low for 8-10 hrs. Then serve.

Equipment Needed:

1. Crockpot

Servings: 4

Preparation Time: 20 minutes
Cooking Time: 10 hours
Total Time: 10 hours

Nutrition Facts

Serving size: 1/4 of a recipe (26.3 ounces).

Amount Per Serving	
Calories	454.89
Calories From Fat (30%)	135.88
	% Daily Value
Total Fat 15.66g	24%
Saturated Fat 6.63g	33%
Cholesterol 74.84mg	25%
Sodium 573.38mg	24%
Potassium 1879.87mg	54%
Total Carbohydrates 53.06g	18%
Fiber 9.3g	37%
Sugar 10.67g	
Protein 29.66g	59%
MyPoints 9.6	

Recipe Tips

Remember you can make this with elk, buffalo or the cheapest cut of beef you can find. Cook it a long time on low heat and it will be tasty and tender.

Chicken Satay

Delicious as an appetizer or main entry! As served at FitBodyRetreat.com.

2	handfuls	sliced chicken, cubed tofu, scallops, shrimp, pork, beef, etc. (about 2 cups)
2	tsp	garlic, chopped
2	tsp	yellow curry powder
1	tsp	Bragg Liquid Aminos
1	tsp	oyster sauce
1	tsp	agave
4	tbsp	macadamia nut oil
1	ea	red pepper

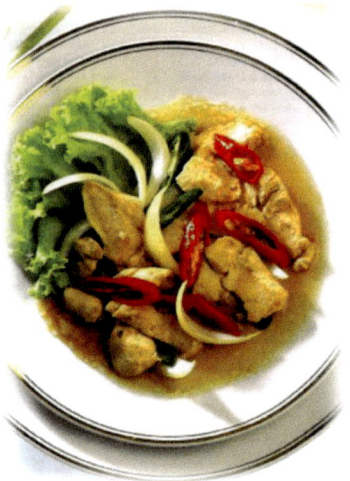

Procedure

1. Mix all ingredients together in a bowl.
2. Fry in a non-stick pan until done.

Servings: 2

Preparation Time: 10 minutes
Cooking Time: 10 minutes
Total Time: 20 minutes

Nutrition Facts

Serving size: 1/2 of a recipe (10.7 ounces).

Amount Per Serving	
Calories	518.5
Calories From Fat (66%)	343.07
	% Daily Value
Total Fat 37.8g	58%
Saturated Fat 2.6g	13%
Cholesterol 105mg	35%
Sodium 275.9mg	11%
Potassium 517.41mg	15%
Total Carbohydrates 6.79g	2%
Fiber 2.26g	9%
Sugar 3.13g	
Protein 36.7g	73%
MyPoints 13.07	

Recipe Tips

I make this dish a lot! It is so easy and so good! You really want to serve it up with a peanut sauce though. Be careful which sauce you buy. Some are high calorie. I use about ½ a teaspoon or 30 calories for my personal use. I learned this dish while kick boxing in Thailand with my oldest son Dan.

Elk Meat Loaf

Jerry Anderson of French Lick taught me this recipe. It's his original version. As served at FitBodyRetreat.com.

10	lbs	ground elk	1/4	cup	sea salt	
10	oz	dried bread crumbs	1	cup	chopped onion	
18	ea	eggs, whole	1	tbsp	black pepper	
1	qt	milk, 2%				

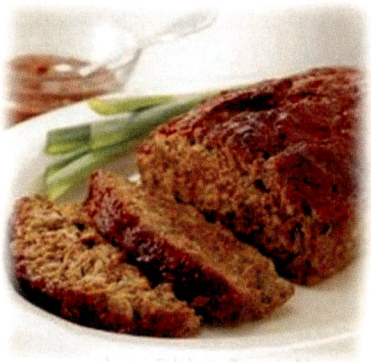

Procedure

1. In a bowl, combine the eggs, onion soup, and bread crumbs.
2. Crumble beef over the mixture and mix well.
3. Shape into a loaf.
4. Place in a greased 11x7x2 baking dish.
5. Bake, uncovered, at 350F for 30 min.
6. Pour mushroom soup over loaf.
7. Bake 1 hr longer or until meat is no longer pink and a meat thermometer reads 180F.
8. Let stand 10 min before slicing.

Servings: 30

Oven Temperature: 350°F

Preparation Time: 20 minutes
Cooking Time: 1 hour and 30 minutes
Total Time: 1 hour and 40 minutes

Nutrition Facts

Serving size: 1/30 of a recipe (8.2 ounces).

Amount Per Serving	
Calories	266.99
Calories From Fat (22%)	58.16
	% Daily Value
Total Fat 6.2g	10%
Saturated Fat 2.27g	11%
Cholesterol 197.36mg	66%
Sodium 1158.13mg	48%
Potassium 588.03mg	17%
Total Carbohydrates 9.21g	3%
Fiber 0.57g	2%
Sugar 2.57g	
Protein 40.88g	82%
MyPoints 5.74	

Recipe Tips

Jerry Anderson and I made heaps of this when we owned a steak house at Elk Ridge, before we opened the Oasis.

Garlic Teriyaki Edamame & Chicken

Another great post workout snack! As served at FitBodyRetreat.com.

1/4	cup	water	1	tbsp	sesame oil
3	ea	garlic cloves, minced	2	tbsp	sesame seeds
16	oz	edamame, frozen (in the pod)	4	ea	chicken breast, cooked (about 2 oz each)
1/8	cup	oyster sauce			
2	tbsp	agave			
2	tbsp	rice vinegar			

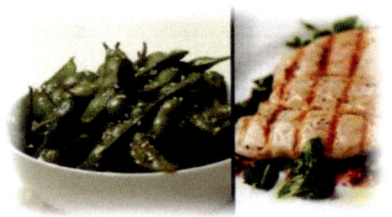

Procedure

1. Bring water and garlic to a boil in a saucepan over high heat.
2. Stir in the edamame and cook until the edamame are hot and the liquid has nearly evaporated, about 5 min.
3. Reduce heat to medium high and stir in oyster sauce, agave, vinegar and sesame oil.
4. Stir constantly until the sauce has thickened and coats the edamame, about 4 min.
5. Sprinkle with sesame seeds.
6. Serve chicken on the side.

Servings: 4

Preparation Time: 10 minutes
Cooking Time: 10 minutes
Total Time: 20 minutes

Nutrition Facts

Serving size: 1/4 of a recipe (12.8 ounces).

Amount Per Serving	
Calories	326.74
Calories From Fat (39%)	126.82
	% Daily Value
Total Fat 13.59g	21%
Saturated Fat 2.08g	10%
Cholesterol 48.2mg	16%
Sodium 310.17mg	13%
Potassium 728.24mg	21%
Total Carbohydrates 17.21g	6%
Fiber 6.5g	26%
Sugar 2.51g	
Protein 30.99g	62%
MyPoints 6.87	

Recipe Tips

More on fat storing: when was the last time you experienced a famine in your life? For most of us - never. But over the past millennium, the earth and its people have experienced many. As a result, our bodies are geared and designed to store fat. Our bodies are designed to prepare for a famine, and it's constantly anticipating being able to survive the next famine through stored fat. So eat right, cheat right, and trick your body! The amazingly effective fat storing device that our body is, can be beat!

Ginger Salmon with Wild Rice

As served at FitBodyRetreat.com.

The Salmon
- 1/2 tsp macadamia nut oil
- 1/4 tsp ginger, freshly grated
- 1 tsp
- 1/2 ea garlic clove, minced
- 1/2 tsp agave
- 4 oz wild salmon

The Rice
- 1/4 cup brown or wild rice mixture
- 1/3 cup vegetable broth, low sodium
- 2 tbsp green onion, sliced 1/4"

The Snow Peas
- 1/2 cup snow peas
- 1/4 tsp lemon pepper

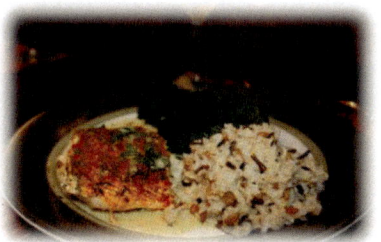

Procedure

The Salmon
1. In a small bowl, combine oil, ginger, garlic and agave, and mix together to create a sauce.
2. Brush sauce on both sides of the salmon and store on a baking sheet in the refrigerator for 20 min.
3. Bake salmon at 350F for about 7 minutes*. Set aside.

The Rice
1. Cook the rice in the vegetable broth instead of water.*

The Snow Peas
1. Steam snow peas lightly if you want them firm.
2. Season to taste with lemon pepper.

Arrangement
1. Create a bed of rice on your plate and serve salmon on top with snow peas.

Servings: 1

Oven Temperature: 350°F

Preparation Time: 10 minutes
Cooking Time: 30 minutes
Total Time: 45 minutes

Nutrition Facts

Serving size: Entire recipe (12.9 ounces).

Amount Per Serving	
Calories	438.61
Calories From Fat (38%)	166.96
	% Daily Value
Total Fat 17.77g	27%
Saturated Fat 2.39g	12%
Cholesterol 132.77mg	44%
Sodium 320.98mg	13%
Potassium 1321.35mg	38%
Total Carbohydrates 13.63g	5%
Fiber 1.92g	8%
Sugar 1.87g	
Protein 51.42g	103%
MyPoints 9.87	

Recipe Tips

If your fat loss and weight loss goals are determined by 80% of what you eat, then shouldn't you be focusing on what goes into your mouth 80% of the time? I find it odd that trainers spend so much time with their clients in the gym and not in the kitchen. At my center, my guests participate in cooking every meal.

* White liquid will rise to the top of the fish when done.

* If you have a rice cooker, use that or follow instructions for cooking on the stove.

Grilled Wasabi Salmon

Tender juicy salmon, served on a bed of rice, quinoa, or wilted spinach and topped with pico-de-gallo. As served at FitBodyRetreat.com.

12	oz	salmon filet	1	squirt	Bragg Liquid Aminos
1	tbsp	macadamia nut oil	1	tsp	wasabi paste
1/4	tsp	black pepper			

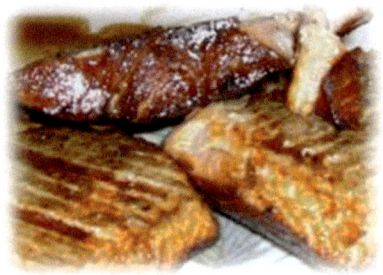

Procedure

1. Preheat grill on high.
2. Lay a piece of tin foil on the grill. Fish has a tendency to fall through the cracks.
3. Rub salmon with oil and sprinkle with pepper.
4. Sear each side 2 min on high starting with skin side down.
5. Turn back over to skin side down.
6. Paint the salmon with a light coating of wasabi paste. The thicker the coating, the hotter the fish.
7. Reduce heat to medium and cook for another 3-5 min.
8. Serve on a bed of rice, quinoa, or wilted spinach and top liquid aminos and pico-de-gallo*.

Servings: 2

Preparation Time: 5 minutes
Cooking Time: 8 minutes
Total Time: 15 minutes

Nutrition Facts

Serving size: 1/2 of a recipe (8.1 ounces).

Amount Per Serving	
Calories	655
Calories From Fat (36%)	237.94
	% Daily Value
Total Fat 26.45g	41%
Saturated Fat 4.41g	22%
Cholesterol 263.66mg	88%
Sodium 144.3mg	6%
Potassium 1636.45mg	47%
Total Carbohydrates 1.17g	<1%
Fiber 0.07g	<1%
Sugar 0g	
Protein 103.14g	206%
MyPoints 15.29	

Recipe Tips

I found this recipe at Timber Line Lodge, a restaurant on Mt. Hood in Oregon. Good stuff!

* See recipe for Pico-de-Gallo.

Lemon Herb Chicken

Citrus adds sparkle to supper with this recipe. Consider replacing the dried herbs in this dish with fresh ones. As served at FitBodyRetreat.com.

8 ea	chicken breast halves, boneless, skinless	
1 ea	lemon, zested	
2 ea	lemons, juiced	
2 tbsp	macadamia nut oil	
2 tsp	dried parsley	
2 tsp	dried chives	
1 tsp	dried thyme	
1/2 tsp	dried oregano	
1/2 tsp	garlic powder	
1/2 tsp	sea salt	
1/2 tsp	black pepper	

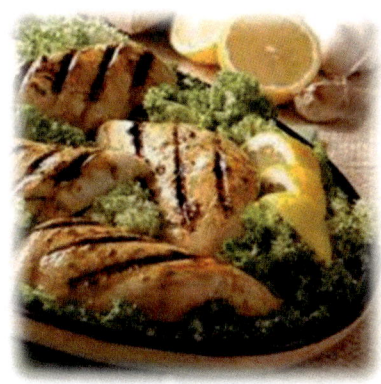

Procedure

1. Rinse chicken and pat dry. Flatten to even thickness.
2. Make a marinade by combining grated lemon peel, lemon juice, macadamia nut oil, parsley, chives, thyme, oregano, garlic, salt and pepper in large flat glass dish or large resealable bag.
3. Add chicken.
4. Turn to coat evenly. Cover. Refrigerate 30 min to 24 hrs, turning occasionally.
5. Prepare grill or heat broiler.
6. Remove chicken from marinade. Then discard marinade.
7. Grill or broil 5 min per side or until chicken is no longer pink in the center.*

Servings: 8

Preparation Time: 20 minutes
Cooking Time: 30 minutes
Total Time: 4 hours

Nutrition Facts

Serving size: 1/8 of a recipe (7.6 ounces).

Amount Per Serving	
Calories	319.44
Calories From Fat (28%)	90.7
	% Daily Value
Total Fat 9.67g	15%
Saturated Fat 1.75g	9%
Cholesterol 146.2mg	49%
Sodium 245.22mg	10%
Potassium 449.45mg	13%
Total Carbohydrates 1.43g	<1%
Fiber 0.17g	<1%
Sugar 0.02g	
Protein 53.44g	107%
MyPoints 7.16	

Recipe Tips

Remember, protein as a snack is far more filling and satisfying than carbs. Plus, you need to have a minimum of ½ gram of protein for every pound you weigh, every day to build muscle and to lose weight. So eat chicken for dinner or a late night snack instead of eating chips or cheese.

* If you prefer, you can bake in oven at 425F for 25 min.

Mediciettes, Steak Appetizer with Bearnaise Sauce

This recipe is yummy and quite simple. It's also adaptable to any personal preferences you may have. We use strictly tenderloin tips in our mediciettes. Bar none, this is my favorite appetizer of all time. We served it at Elk Ridge when we owned a steak house. The recipe is originally from a small family owned restaurant in Lancing, Michigan, called the Nite Cap. The chef responsible for this recipe is Carl J. Davis. As served at FitBodyRetreat.com.

1	lb	tenderloin tips	1	tbsp	parsley
1/4	cup	Wishbone Italian dressing	1/2	tbsp	parmesan cheese
1	cup	Panko bread crumbs			Non-stick cooking spray

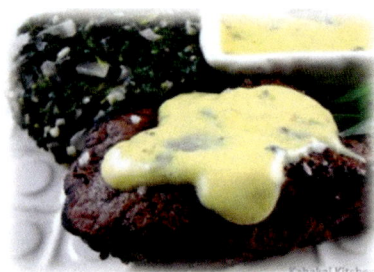

Procedure

1. Cut up tenderloin tips into about 1oz pieces.
2. Place these in the Italian dressing for 2+ hrs to marinate. We use Wishbone for consistency.
3. Roll the steak pieces in the Panko bread crumbs with parsley and parmesan mixture.
4. Spray cookie sheet with non-stick spray.
5. Bake these on a cookie sheet at 400F for about 8-10 min or until browned.
6. Serve this dish with bearnaise sauce*. Just dip the pieces in the sauce and enjoy!

Servings: 4

Oven Temperature: 400°F

Preparation Time: 20 minutes
Cooking Time: 12 minutes
Total Time: 45 minutes

Nutrition Facts

Serving size: 1/4 of a recipe (5.4 ounces).

Amount Per Serving	
Calories	366.35
Calories From Fat (70%)	255.88
	% Daily Value
Total Fat 27.96g	43%
Saturated Fat 11.05g	55%
Cholesterol 81.06mg	27%
Sodium 153.59mg	6%
Potassium 352.39mg	10%
Total Carbohydrates 5.89g	2%
Fiber 0.31g	1%
Sugar 0.58g	
Protein 21.27g	43%
MyPoints 9.6	

Recipe Tips

Take heed when serving up this dish. It is so damn good your friends will keep coming over for more! And don't even bother serving this without the sauce! It's so easy to make! Note: Not approved unless a cheat day!

*See the Béarnaise Sauce II recipe in this book.

Perfect Filet Mignon

Taught to me at a classy restaurant in Boston! As served at FitBodyRetreat.com.

4	6 oz	filet mignon steaks	1	dash	cracked black pepper (to taste)
4	tsp	Bragg Liquid Aminos	4	tbsp	macadamia nut oil

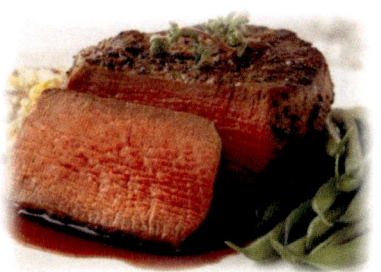

Procedure

1. Place steaks on a rack where they can get air and come up to room temperature (about an hour).
2. Season or paint steaks with liquid aminos.
3. Paint steaks with oil.
4. Sprinkle them with pepper.
5. Heat a good frying pan on high for at least 3 min.
6. With tongs, place steaks into pan.
7. Cook for 2-1/2 min, then turn and cook for another 2-1/2 min.
8. Remove steaks from the pan immediately and place them back on the rack for an hour or more.
9. Heat oven to 425F.
10. Place steaks back into the pan you seared them in.
11. Place the pan in the oven.
12. Cooking times: 8 min for rare; 10 min for med; 12 min for well done.

Servings: 4

Oven Temperature: 425°F

Preparation Time: 15 minutes
Cooking Time: 15 minutes
Total Time: 1 hour

Nutrition Facts

Serving size: 1/4 of a recipe (1.7 ounces).

Amount Per Serving	
Calories	176.76
Calories From Fat (80%)	141.27
	% Daily Value
Total Fat 16.38g	25%
Saturated Fat 0.91g	5%
Cholesterol 23.25mg	8%
Sodium 177.01mg	7%
Potassium 105.23mg	3%
Total Carbohydrates 0.02g	<1%
Fiber 0.01g	<1%
Sugar 0g	
Protein 9.24g	18%
MyPoints 4.9	

Recipe Tips

If calories are not an issue, top each steak with a fat slice of butter and a pinch of sea salt to melt away! It may seem complicated, but it's really not! While at a telecom conference in Boston, I went into the kitchen of the Palm Restaurant. I thought I was an expert at preparing "the perfect steak". This, my friend, is how they taught me to make the perfect steak! Note: At the Palm, they use sea salt, pepper and olive oil. This is my version of their perfect fillet.

Pork Tenderloin

Juicy and delicious! Tastes great sliced on a sandwich or with eggs in the morning. As served at FitBodyRetreat.com.

4 lbs pork tenderloin, whole   herbs of your choice

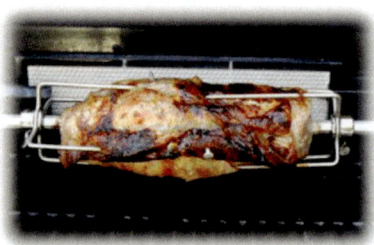

Procedure

1. Place tenderloin on the rotisserie.
2. Set the timer for 17 min per lb. or 68 min to be exact. (the machine calls for 18 min per lb).
3. When it stops, take it out and slice it up.

Equipment Needed:

1. Ronco Rotisserie

Servings: 10

Preparation Time: 5 minutes
Cooking Time: 1 hour and 8 minutes
Total Time: 1 hour and 15 minutes

Nutrition Facts

Serving size: 1/10 of a recipe (4.7 ounces).

Amount Per Serving	
Calories	190.61
Calories From Fat (23%)	44.18
	% Daily Value
Total Fat 4.68g	7%
Saturated Fat 1.6g	8%
Cholesterol 97.24mg	32%
Sodium 75.95mg	3%
Potassium 562.54mg	16%
Total Carbohydrates 0.02g	<1%
Fiber 0.01g	<1%
Sugar 0g	
Protein 34.88g	70%
MyPoints 4.2	

Recipe Tips

I'd guess I've owned 4 of these Ronco rotisserie machines over the years. You can find them on eBay for about $50. You cannot screw up a piece of meat on these things. They work amazingly well!

Prime Rib Tenderloin

Another simple easy dish that will knock your socks off! As served at FitBodyRetreat.com.

4 lbs   beef loin, whole   herbs of your choice

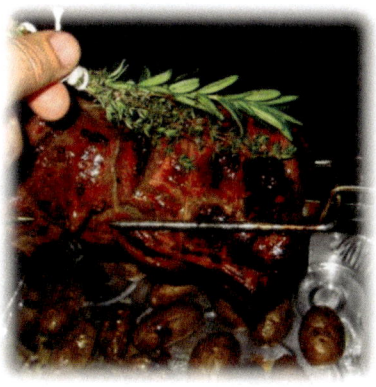

Procedure

1. Rub meat with herbs of your choice.
2. Place it in the rotisserie at 17 min per lb. or 68 minutes to be exact.
3. When done, take it out, slice it thin and serve.

Equipment Needed:

1. Ronco Rotisserie

Servings: 8

Preparation Time: 5 minutes
Cooking Time: 1 hour and 8 minutes
Total Time: 1 hour and 15 minutes

Nutrition Facts

Serving size: 1/8 of a recipe (8 ounces).

Amount Per Serving	
Calories	644.28
Calories From Fat (74%)	478.89
	% Daily Value
Total Fat 52.3g	80%
Saturated Fat 21.48g	107%
Cholesterol 158.76mg	53%
Sodium 108.89mg	5%
Potassium 678.08mg	19%
Total Carbohydrates 0.02g	<1%
Fiber 0.01g	<1%
Sugar 0g	
Protein 40.62g	81%
MyPoints 17.24	

Recipe Tips

Be careful about making this taste too good! Like any method of eating, there is poor, good, and then there is extreme. Just treat your food as fuel or fun, and you will do fine. I'd call this dish a bit extreme -- simply because I know it's so good, I'm going to want to eat 3 servings of it!

Quinoa Curry & Chicken

A favorite side dish at the ranch. As served at DetoxOasis.net.

1/2	cup	quinoa	1	tsp	yellow curry powder (heaping tsp)
1/2	tbsp	macadamia nut oil (or olive oil)	1/4	tsp	cinnamon
1-3/4	cup	water	1/2	cup	frozen peas (or fresh)
1/2	ea	onion, diced (about 4-5 oz)	4	oz	chicken breast, cooked
1	tsp	fresh ginger root, grated	1/4	cup	cheddar cheese, shredded, reduced fat
1	tsp	turmeric (heaping tsp)			

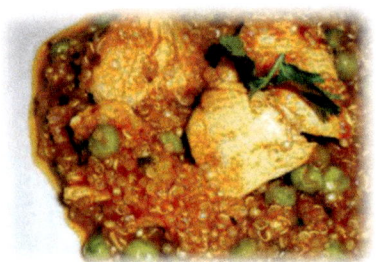

Procedure

1. Add quinoa, water and oil to a saucepan and bring to a boil.
2. Simmer for 20 min.
3. Add onion, ginger root, turmeric, curry, cinnamon and peas and heat through.
4. Place quinoa mixture on a plate.
5. Place cooked chicken breast on top of quinoa.
6. Melt cheese on top and serve.

Servings: 6

Preparation Time: 5 minutes
Cooking Time: 20 minutes
Total Time: 30 minutes

Nutrition Facts

Serving size: 1/6 of a recipe (4.6 ounces).

Amount Per Serving	
Calories	117.05
Calories From Fat (24%)	28.64
	% Daily Value
Total Fat 3.17g	5%
Saturated Fat 0.53g	3%
Cholesterol 17.05mg	6%
Sodium 58.42mg	2%
Potassium 180.15mg	5%
Total Carbohydrates 12.23g	4%
Fiber 1.92g	8%
Sugar 1.04g	
Protein 9.79g	20%
MyPoints 2.22	

Recipe Tips

About turmeric -- See what happens when I get clients from the Middle East at our retreat center! I need a few more clients from South America to help me expand my food knowledge. Funny, I have a client from France; she comes every 60 days and yet I have learned no French cooking! What's with that Marie?

Raw-Zucchini Pasta

A simple pasta alternative with our Spaghetti Sauce or Raw Alfredo Sauce. As served at DetoxOasis.net.

1 ea zucchini, raw

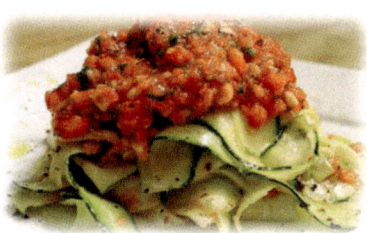

Procedure

1. Peel the skin off the zucchini with a vegetable peeler.
2. Peel the zucchini down to the seeds.
3. Place the peelings in a bowl.
4. Serve with our Spaghetti Sauce or Raw Alfredo Sauce.

Servings: 1

Preparation Time: 5 minutes
Cooking Time: 5 minutes
Total Time: 5 minutes

Nutrition Facts

Serving size: Entire recipe (6.9 ounces).

Amount Per Serving	
Calories	33.32
Calories From Fat (16%)	5.33
	% Daily Value
Total Fat 0.63g	<1%
Saturated Fat 0.16g	<1%
Cholesterol 0mg	0%
Sodium 15.68mg	<1%
Potassium 511.56mg	15%
Total Carbohydrates 6.1g	2%
Fiber 1.96g	8%
Sugar 4.9g	
Protein 2.37g	5%
MyPoints 0.33	

Recipe Tips

I love raw foods! But I also eat a balance of cooked foods. My rule of thumb is this: when I meet someone who looks amazing, I like to ask them about their diet. It is the person that looks amazing that you will learn the most from regarding how you, too, may improve your diet and your look! Take a look at the raw foodie Jenna Norwood down Sarasota way. She's quite possibly one of the fittest and sexiest raw ladies out there. She has some amazing videos and books published. Check out her work. Kelly Serbonich, former chef at Hippocrates Institute in South Florida, first introduced me to raw pasta here at my ranch in Indiana. Together, we did a short local television show on raw foods.

Salmon & Cucumber Quinoa Salad

As served at FitBodyRetreat.com.

1	tbsp	rice wine vinegar	1	cup	cucumber, chopped, with skin
1	tsp	macadamia nut oil	2	oz	salmon, cooked
1/2	tsp	sesame oil, toasted	1/2	cup	quinoa, cooked*
1	tsp	Bragg Liquid Aminos	1	tsp	sesame seeds
1/4	tsp	cayenne pepper			

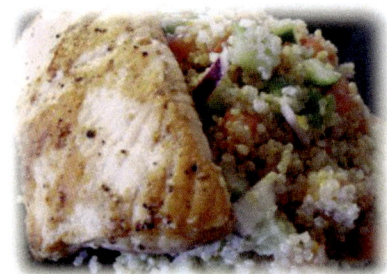

Procedure

1. Combine vinegar, macadamia nut oil, sesame oil, liquid aminos and cayenne pepper in a medium size bowl.
2. Add the cucumber, salmon, quinoa and sesame seeds.
3. Mix well and serve.

Servings: 1

Preparation Time: 10 minutes
Cooking Time: 15 minutes
Total Time: 30 minutes

Nutrition Facts

Serving size: Entire recipe (12.3 ounces).

Amount Per Serving	
Calories	377.73
Calories From Fat (40%)	152.45
	% Daily Value
Total Fat 18.07g	28%
Saturated Fat 1.74g	9%
Cholesterol 66.39mg	22%
Sodium 223.03mg	9%
Potassium 1057.4mg	30%
Total Carbohydrates 29.85g	10%
Fiber 4g	16%
Sugar 1.89g	
Protein 30.23g	60%
MyPoints 8.26	

Recipe Tips

Food is either fuel or fun. Rarely is it both! Treat each meal as fuel, and you will reach your goals much faster. The food fun starts after you reach your body fat and weight goals! Though this dish is pretty good fun for the amount of fuel!

* See recipe for Quinoa Basic.

Seared Ahi Tuna

Tender tuna served on a bed of rice, quinoa, or wilted spinach and topped with pico-de-gallo. As served at FitBodyRetreat.com.

12	oz	tuna steak	1/4	tsp	black pepper
1	tbsp	macadamia nut oil	1	squirt	Bragg Liquid Aminos

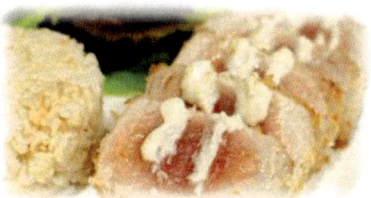

Procedure

1. Preheat skillet on a high heat.
2. Rub tuna with oil and sprinkle with black pepper.
3. Sear each side for 2 min on high,
4. Place a cover on the pan.
5. Reduce heat to medium and cook another 3-5 min.
6. Serve on a bed of rice, quinoa, or wilted spinach and top with liquid aminos and our pico-de-gallo* if you'd like.

Servings: 2

Preparation Time: 5 minutes
Cooking Time: 8 minutes
Total Time: 15 minutes

Nutrition Facts

Serving size: 1/2 of a recipe (8 ounces).

Amount Per Serving	
Calories	373.46
Calories From Fat (44%)	163.58
	% Daily Value
Total Fat 17.68g	27%
Saturated Fat 2.74g	14%
Cholesterol 83.3mg	28%
Sodium 95.05mg	4%
Potassium 552.59mg	16%
Total Carbohydrates 0.17g	<1%
Fiber 0.07g	<1%
Sugar 0g	
Protein 50.87g	102%
MyPoints 8.93	

Recipe Tips

Saturday comes only once a week! Every night can't be Saturday night. Abuse your body once a week with party food and drink, and you will do fine. I like to top my tuna with a horseradish lite mayo sauce.

* See recipe for Pico-de-Gallo.

Shrimp & Rice Penne Pasta

Wheat and gluten free. As served at FitBodyRetreat.com.

2	tbsp	macadamia nut oil	1	med	zucchini, chopped
12	oz	shrimp, peeled and deveined	4	ea	Roma tomatoes, seeded and chopped
1	tsp	Bragg Liquid Aminos	1/4	cup	fresh basil, chopped (or 1 tsp dried)
1	tsp	extra virgin olive oil			
1	cup	pasta, rice penne, dry*	1/4	tsp	black pepper freshly ground
1	ea	garlic clove, minced			
1	med	Italian eggplant, peeled, and cut in 1/2" cubes	1	tbsp	Parmesan cheese

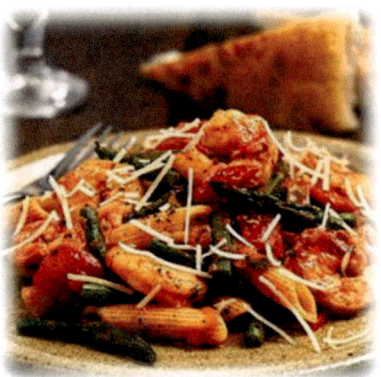

Procedure

1. Heat 1 tbsp of macadamia nut oil in pan and stir-fry the shrimp until done. Set aside.
2. Boil water for pasta in a medium size pot.
3. When water starts to boil, add liquid aminos and tsp of olive oil.
4. Add rice pasta to the water and cook according to directions.
5. While pasta is cooking, heat remaining macadamia nut oil in large skillet.
6. Sauté garlic for 1 minute.
7. Add eggplant and zucchini and sauté for 5 minutes or until a nice brown.
8. Add chopped tomatoes and sauté for an additional 2 minutes.
9. Add shrimp back to pan and cook for another 2 minutes until shrimp are cooked through.
10. Drain pasta and toss all ingredients together.
11. Top the pasta with chopped basil.
12. Add fresh ground pepper and parmesan cheese (about 1 tsp per serving).

Servings: 4

Preparation Time: 15 minutes
Cooking Time: 30 minutes
Total Time: 1 hour

Nutrition Facts

Serving size: 1/4 of a recipe (14.4 ounces).

Amount Per Serving		
Calories		294.85
Calories From Fat (31%)		92.53
		% Daily Value
Total Fat 10.7g		16%
Saturated Fat 0.58g		3%
Cholesterol 108.26mg		36%
Sodium 552.3mg		23%
Potassium 774.76mg		22%
Total Carbohydrates 34.97g		12%
Fiber 5.92g		24%
Sugar 7.05g		
Protein 17.67g		35%
MyPoints 5.99		

Recipe Tips

I rarely eat pasta. But when I do, it's rice pasta and there is red wine involved.

* We use Tinkyada Brown Rice Penne Pasta with Rice Bran at our center.

Spaghetti Squash with Chicken Breast

The strands of a baked spaghetti squash are tossed with feta cheese, sautéed vegetables, olives, and basil. As served at FitbodyRetreat.com.

1	ea	squash, spaghetti (halved lengthwise and seeded)	1	ea	chicken breast (4 oz)	
2	tbsp	macadamia nut oil	1-1/2	cups	tomatoes, chopped	
1	ea	onion, chopped	3/4	cup	feta cheese, crumbled	
1	ea	garlic clove, minced	3	tbsp	black olives, sliced	
			2	tbsp	fresh basil, chopped	

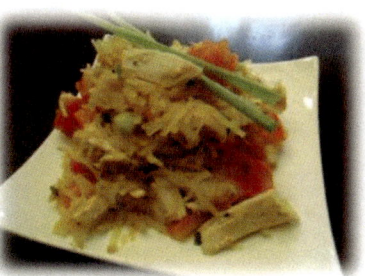

Procedure

1. Preheat oven to 350F (175C).
2. Lightly grease a baking sheet.
3. Place spaghetti squash cut sides down on the prepared baking sheet and bake for 30 min in preheated oven, or until a sharp knife can be inserted with minimal resistance.
4. Remove squash from oven and set aside to cool enough to be easily handled.
5. Cook chicken either in oven or on a grill.
6. Heat oil in a skillet over medium heat.
7. Sauté onion in oil until tender.
8. Add garlic and sauté for 2-3 min.
9. Stir in tomatoes and cook only until tomatoes are warm. Set aside.
10. Use a large spoon to scoop the stringy pulp from the squash and place in medium bowl.
11. Toss with the sautéed vegetables, feta cheese and basil.
12. Top with sliced chicken breast.
13. Serve warm.

Servings: 6

Oven Temperature: 350°F

Preparation Time: 15 minutes
Cooking Time: 30 minutes
Total Time: 45 minutes

Nutrition Facts

Serving size: 1/6 of a recipe (5.2 ounces).

Amount Per Serving	
Calories	162.09
Calories From Fat (53%)	86.66
	% Daily Value
Total Fat 10.12g	16%
Saturated Fat 3.01g	15%
Cholesterol 28.78mg	10%
Sodium 288.68mg	12%
Potassium 292.21mg	8%
Total Carbohydrates 11.55g	4%
Fiber 1.3g	5%
Sugar 3.82g	
Protein 8.27g	17%
MyPoints 3.83	

Recipe Tips

What I really like about spaghetti squash is its texture, flavor, and lack of calories. I like to top it with coconut oil and cinnamon.

Thai-Garlic Chicken

Simple and tasty! As served at FitBodyRetreat.com.

2	handfuls	chicken breast, thinly sliced (about 2 cups)	1	tsp	Bragg Liquid Aminos
2	tsp	garlic, chopped	1	tsp	agave
1	tsp	oyster sauce	1/8	tsp	white pepper
			2	tsp	macadamia nut oil

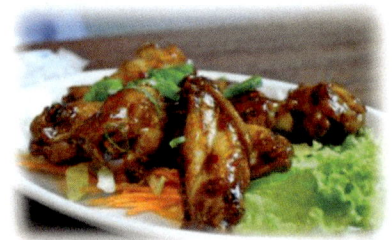

Procedure

1. Mix all ingredients together except for the oil.
2. Add oil to non-stick pan on medium heat.
3. Add all ingredients to pan and cook until done.

Servings: 1

Preparation Time: 10 minutes
Cooking Time: 10 minutes
Total Time: 20 minutes

Nutrition Facts

Serving size: Entire recipe (14.5 ounces).

Amount Per Serving	
Calories	435.48
Calories From Fat (37%)	160.63
	% Daily Value
Total Fat 16.72g	26%
Saturated Fat 1.62g	8%
Cholesterol 181.44mg	60%
Sodium 662.8mg	28%
Potassium 1074.86mg	31%
Total Carbohydrates 2.71g	<1%
Fiber 0.21g	<1%
Sugar 0.06g	
Protein 61.66g	123%
MyPoints 10.06	

Recipe Tips

I don't care whether it's wings, breasts or thighs, or whatever other part of the chicken you choose. This will be a favorite recipe! Pork works well with this recipe too.

Thai-Spicy Easy Fish

Hot and spicy. Easy to make. As served at FitBodyRetreat.com.

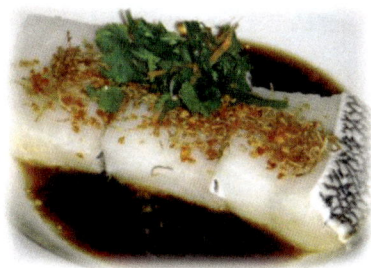

The Base
1	ea	cod fillet (or any white fish)
1	tsp	macadamia nut oil
1/2	tbsp	green curry
2	tsp	garlic, chopped
1	tsp	oyster sauce
1	tsp	Bragg Liquid Aminos
1	tsp	agave
1	tsp	white pepper

The Sauce
4	tsp	water
2	tsp	agave
2	tsp	fish sauce
2	tsp	oyster sauce
2	tsp	lemon juice
1	tsp	macadamia nut oil

Procedure
1. Place fish and oil in a non-stick pan with the green curry.
2. Add remaining ingredients to pan, except for sauce, and mix well.
3. Mix sauce ingredients in a separate bowl.
4. Place fish on 1/2 the sauce, and place remaining 1/2 of sauce on top of fish.

Servings: 1

Preparation Time: 10 minutes
Cooking Time: 10 minutes
Total Time: 20 minutes

Nutrition Facts
Serving size: Entire recipe (23.4 ounces).

Amount Per Serving	
Calories	365.48
Calories From Fat (32%)	118.49
	% Daily Value
Total Fat 11.03g	17%
Saturated Fat 0.33g	2%
Cholesterol 99.33mg	33%
Sodium 1997.47mg	83%
Potassium 1033.18mg	30%
Total Carbohydrates 8.1g	3%
Fiber 0.83g	3%
Sugar 0.75g	
Protein 43.63g	87%
MyPoints 8.06	

Recipe Tips
If you notice the ingredients, almost all Thai dishes contain the same stuff!

Turkey & Fruit

Turkey breast and fruit - just right for the post workout feeding! As served at FitBodyRetreat.com.

- 2 oz turkey breast, grilled (or chicken)
- 1/4 cup apple, sliced
- 1/4 cup mandarin orange
- 1/4 ea ruby red grapefruit
- 1/4 cup blueberries

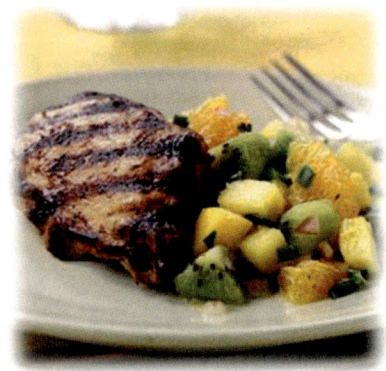

Procedure

1. Slice up fruit and put into a cup.
2. Serve with protein. Can substitute any meat - chicken, buffalo, fish, etc..

Servings: 1

Preparation Time: 10 minutes
Cooking Time:
Total Time: 15 minutes

Nutrition Facts

Serving size: Entire recipe (6 ounces).

Amount Per Serving	
Calories	166.96
Calories From Fat (23%)	38.42
	% Daily Value
Total Fat 4.44g	7%
Saturated Fat 1.22g	6%
Cholesterol 41.96mg	14%
Sodium 38.32mg	2%
Potassium 299.51mg	9%
Total Carbohydrates 16.37g	5%
Fiber 4.5g	18%
Sugar 9.08g	
Protein 17.05g	34%
MyPoints 2.91	

Recipe Tips

I sometimes get complaints at my center about not offering enough fruit in my recipes. Here you go!

Wasabi Salmon

This spicy salmon filet may be grilled, smoked with apple chips, or roasted in the oven.

3 lbs	salmon filet	Non-stick cooking spray
1 tbsp	wasabi powder	

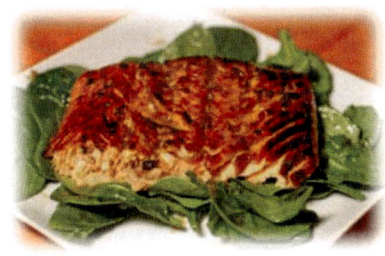

Procedure

1. Preheat oven to 400F (200C).
2. Spray baking sheet with non-stick cooking spray.
3. Place the salmon, skin side down, on baking sheet.
4. Bake for 10 min in the oven, or until fish flakes with a fork.
5. Spread the wasabi powder on top of the filet after 10 min.
6. Cook another 10 min.

Servings: 8

Oven Temperature: 400°F

Preparation Time: 10 minutes
Cooking Time: 20 minutes
Total Time: 30 minutes

Nutrition Facts

Serving size: 1/8 of a recipe (6.5 ounces).

Amount Per Serving	
Calories	587.95
Calories From Fat (30%)	174.86
	% Daily Value
Total Fat 19.45g	30%
Saturated Fat 4.41g	22%
Cholesterol 263.66mg	88%
Sodium 86.92mg	4%
Potassium 1638.73mg	47%
Total Carbohydrates 0.24g	<1%
Fiber 0.08g	<1%
Sugar 0g	
Protein 103.16g	206%
MyPoints 13.36	

Sides

Oasis Lodging

When possible, add grain side dishes before 6pm. Generally, a ½ cup serving is all you need, except in regards to quinoa, whereas a ¼ cup is all you will need. The calories in quinoa are quite high.

Although we only have just a few veggie recipes here, it's simply because they are our favorites.   Follow this rule of thumb, if it's green then you can has much of it as you like.

Dinner served at the Oasis after the initial 6 day detox looks like this:

    4 to 6 ounces of protein: either… fish, tofu, elk, beef, turkey, chicken, or bison
    Either: ½ cup of wild rice, or ¼ cup quinoa, or ½ sweet potato, or black beans, or lentils
    Anything green: spinach salad, asparagus, broccoli, or green salad

    Note the word "either" above; it's not all of the above but one selection from each group!
    Our Oasis goal of 325 to 400 calories for the dinner meal

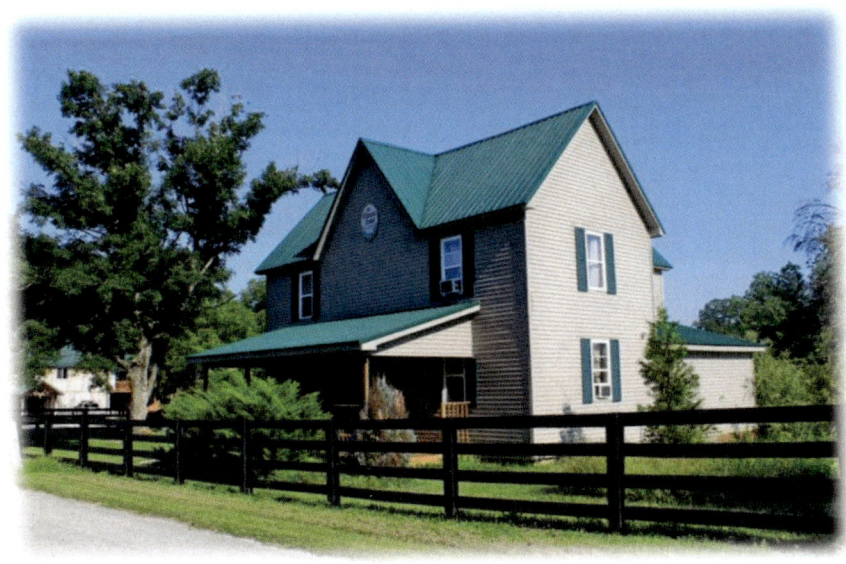

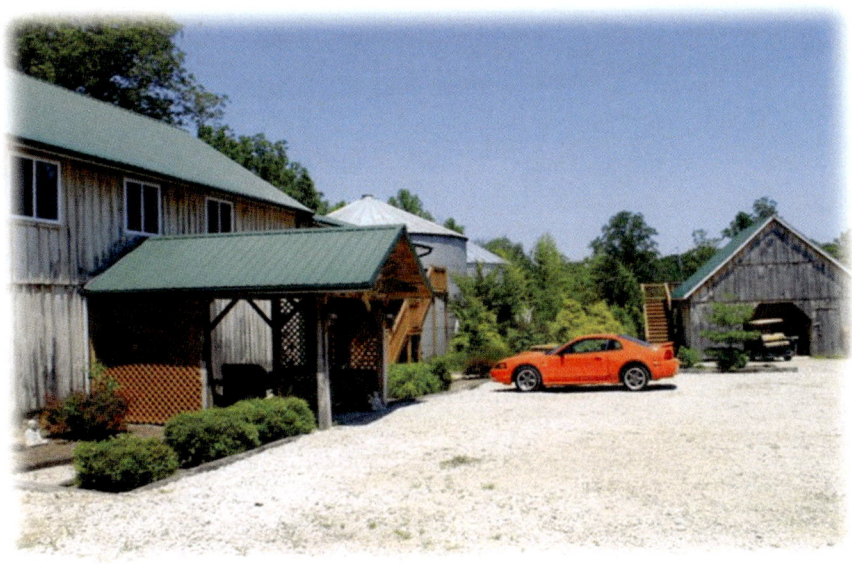

Asparagus (vegetable)

A great tasting vegetable that goes well with any meal. As served at FitBodyRetreat.com.

1	bunch	asparagus (about 10 stalks)	1 squirt	Bragg Liquid Aminos (optional)

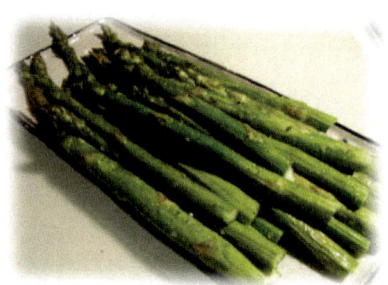

Procedure

1. Heat water to a boil.
2. Cut ends off of asparagus before adding to water.
3. Simmer for 6-8 min.
4. Pull them out while still firm.
5. Season with liquid aminos and serve.

Servings: 4

Preparation Time: 5 minutes
Cooking Time: 10 minutes
Total Time: 15 minutes

Nutrition Facts

Serving size: 1/4 of a recipe (1.8 ounces).

Amount Per Serving	
Calories	6.75
Calories From Fat (0%)	0
	% Daily Value
Total Fat 0g	0%
Sodium 5.75mg	<1%
Total Carbohydrates 1.25g	<1%
Protein 0.75g	2%
MyPoints 0.14	

Recipe Tips

Every night for dinner you need a green. I do this: any meat - any green - any bean or wild grain.

Black Beans Basic (legume)

Just beans and an onion. As served at FitBodyRetreat.com.

16	oz	black beans, fresh (soaked overnight)	1	ea	onion, sliced
6	cups	water	1	tbsp	macadamia nut oil (or olive oil)

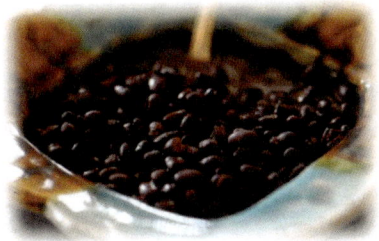

Procedure

1. Drain and rinse beans.
2. Place beans, water, onions and oil into a saucepan and bring to a boil.
3. Simmer for 1-1/2 to 2 hrs. Then serve.*

Servings: 9

Preparation Time: 10 minutes
Cooking Time: 2 hours
Total Time: 2 hours and 10 minutes

Nutrition Facts

Serving size: 1/9 of a recipe (7.9 ounces).

Amount Per Serving	
Calories	85.43
Calories From Fat (17%)	14.41
	% Daily Value
Total Fat 1.57g	2%
Saturated Fat 0.01g	<1%
Cholesterol 0mg	0%
Sodium 5.28mg	<1%
Potassium 21.41mg	<1%
Total Carbohydrates 13.71g	5%
Fiber 0.23g	<1%
Sugar 0.58g	
Protein 3.7g	7%
MyPoints 1.79	

Recipe Tips

I eat a lot of beans, lentils and quinoa. Remember this -- 1/2 cup of beans and lentils is all you need and only 1/8 cup of quinoa. Why? Look at the calorie counts on these foods! With quinoa, I freeze it up in ½ or ¼ cup. Then, when I pull it out of the freezer and zap it in a microwave for 2 minutes, it's good to go. Again, like the chicken breasts prepared in advance, if it's ready to eat, then you can eat clean and good. That's the problem with fast food or processed food, it's ready when we want it. Try and make your healthy food items ahead of time so they're ready when you want them. Plan ahead just a bit and you will succeed. If it's already cooked and in your freezer, you will be more likely to eat it, simply because it's already prepared and can be ready in 5 minutes. When you're hungry, your patience to wait for food is compromised! It's at this time that we tend to make poor eating choices. Plan ahead and you will do fine.

* For flavor, add Bragg Liquid Aminos and a pinch of parsley for color.

Brown Rice (grain)

Just some good carbs here! Serving size is 1/2 cup. As served at FitBodyRetreat.com.

1 cup brown rice
2-1/2 cup water
1/4 tsp extra virgin olive oil

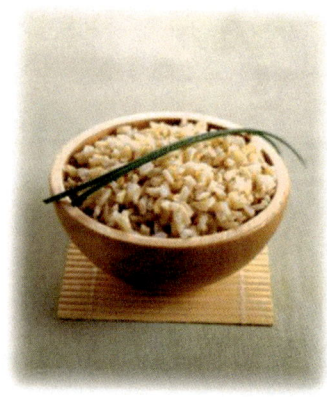

Procedure

1. Add water, rice and oil to saucepan.*
2. Bring water to a boil, then simmer for about 45 min.
3. Cook until all water is absorbed.

Servings: 7

Preparation Time: 5 minutes
Cooking Time: 45 minutes
Total Time: 1 hour

Nutrition Facts

Serving size: 1/7 of a recipe (4 ounces).

Amount Per Serving	
Calories	98.56
Calories From Fat (9%)	8.49
	% Daily Value
Total Fat 1.02g	2%
Saturated Fat 0.02g	<1%
Cholesterol 0mg	0%
Sodium 2.54mg	<1%
Potassium 0.85mg	<1%
Total Carbohydrates 22.86g	8%
Fiber 1.71g	7%
Sugar 0g	
Protein 1.71g	3%
MyPoints 1.71	

Recipe Tips

Follow instructions on rice bag. Generally when using the rice cooker, you may need to add an extra 1/8 or 1/4 cup more water than the instructions suggest. With most rice, it's a 2 to 1 ratio (2 cups of water per every cup of rice). I eat a lot of beans, lentils, quinoa and WILD RICE! A ½ cup will set you right! Mix with beans and you have some serious muscle fuel. Remember this ½ cup of rice is all you need. If quinoa, a 1/8 cup. Quinoa is high on the calorie side. Personally, I freeze it up in ½ cup. A 2 minute zap in a microwave and it's good to go. Again, like the chicken breasts cooked up in advance, if it's ready to eat, then you can eat clean and good. That's the problem with fast food or processed food. It's ready when we want it. Make your good choices ready when you want them. Plan ahead just a bit and you will succeed. The people I work with that actually write down or record what they eat, have a 200% better success rate in reaching their body fat and weight loss goals than those that do not write or track their the foods they eat. At our retreat center, we use Fitday.com for tracking. It's fast, free and easy to use.

* If using a rice cooker, add all ingredients and press brown rice option until done.

Coconut Sweet Potato or Yam (vegetable)

Tasty baked yams that go with any dish! As served at FitBodyRetreat.com.

1	ea	sweet potato, large	1/2	tsp	cinnamon
1/2	tsp	extra virgin coconut oil			

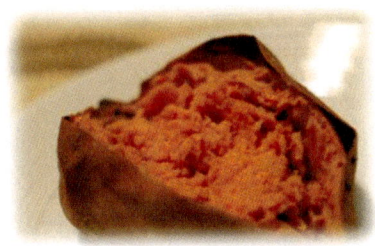

Procedure

1. Wrap the potato in tin foil.*
2. Bake in oven at 425F for 45 min.
3. Remove from oven and cut in half.
4. Drizzle some coconut oil onto it and sprinkle with cinnamon. Then serve.

Servings: 2

Oven Temperature: 425°F

Preparation Time: 5 minutes
Cooking Time: 45 minutes
Total Time: 1 hour

Nutrition Facts

Serving size: 1/2 of a recipe (2.4 ounces).

Amount Per Serving	
Calories	67.2
Calories From Fat (15%)	10.24
	% Daily Value
Total Fat 1.17g	2%
Saturated Fat 0.99g	5%
Cholesterol 0mg	0%
Sodium 35.82mg	1%
Potassium 221.85mg	6%
Total Carbohydrates 13.6g	5%
Fiber 2.3g	9%
Sugar 2.73g	
Protein 1.05g	2%
MyPoints 0.98	

Recipe Tips

It does not get any easier than this. Remember when I said any green, any meat, and bean or wild rice? You can serve this up in place of your rice now and again!

* For extra flavor, first rub the yam with olive oil and sea salt before you wrap it up in foil.

Forbidden Black Wild Rice (grain)

Just a spoonful of black rice bran contains more health promoting anthocyanin antioxidants than are found in a spoonful of blueberries, but with less sugar and more fiber and vitamin E antioxidants. As served at FitBodyRetreat.com.

2	cup	wild black rice	1/2	tsp	Bragg Liquid Aminos
4	cup	water	1/4	tsp	extra virgin olive oil

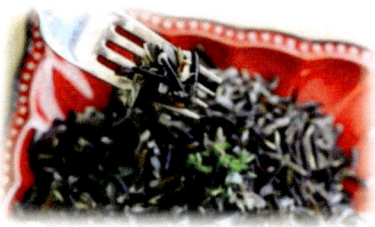

Procedure

1. Put rice in a metal sieve and rinse with cold water.
2. Place rice in a medium sauce pan, cover with cold water and let soak overnight.
3. Drain rice through the sieve.
4. Return rice to the sauce pan and add water, liquid aminos and oil.
5. Bring contents to a boil over high heat.
6. Cover pan with tight lid and reduce heat to low.
7. Simmer rice for 20 minutes. Check texture - should be soft yet chewy. If rice feels too tough, replace lid and cook for 5-10 min more.

Servings: 14

Preparation Time: 5 minutes
Cooking Time: 1 hour and 30 minutes
Total Time: 2 hours

Nutrition Facts

Serving size: 1/14 of a recipe (3.2 ounces).

Amount Per Serving	
Calories	82.31
Calories From Fat (3%)	2.87
	% Daily Value
Total Fat 0.33g	<1%
Saturated Fat 0.05g	<1%
Cholesterol 0mg	0%
Sodium 9.35mg	<1%
Potassium 98.28mg	3%
Total Carbohydrates 17.12g	6%
Fiber 1.42g	6%
Sugar 0.57g	
Protein 3.4g	7%
MyPoints 1.39	

Recipe Tips

If you prefer using a rice cooker, add all ingredients and hit the white rice option until it shuts off. We cook the hard red rice the same way.

Green Beans (legume)

Green beans as a side dish. As served at FitBodyRetreat.com.

2 lbs fresh green beans
1 squirt Bragg Liquid Aminos (optional)

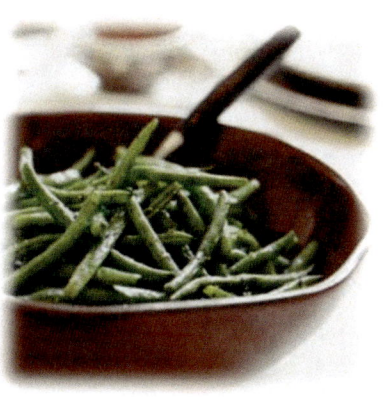

Procedure

1. Heat water to a boil.
2. Cut off stems from beans before adding to water.
3. Simmer for 6-8 min.
4. Pull them out while still firm.
5. Season with liquid aminos and serve.

Servings: 6

Preparation Time: 5 minutes
Cooking Time: 5 minutes
Total Time: 10 minutes

Nutrition Facts

Serving size: 1/6 of a recipe (5.9 ounces).

Amount Per Serving	
Calories	46.87
Calories From Fat (5%)	2.48
	% Daily Value
Total Fat 0.33g	<1%
Saturated Fat 0.08g	<1%
Cholesterol 0mg	0%
Sodium 12.41mg	<1%
Potassium 319.03mg	9%
Total Carbohydrates 10.54g	4%
Fiber 4.08g	16%
Sugar 4.93g	
Protein 2.77g	6%
MyPoints 0.16	

Recipe Tips

Remember – Bragg Liquid Aminos is a great substitute for salt. Any recipe that calls for a teaspoon of salt, I substitute the same amount of Braggs.

Himalayan Red Rice (grain)

The flavor of red rice has been described as nutty and earthy. In addition to being flavorful, the rice is quite aromatic. As served at FitBodyRetreat.com.

1/4	tsp	extra virgin olive oil	2	cup	water
1	cup	red rice	1	tbsp	Bragg Liquid Aminos

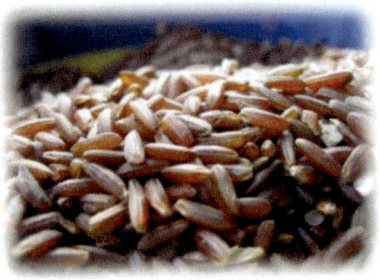

Procedure

1. In a large saucepan, heat oil.*
2. Add rice and cook on high heat, stirring constantly until lightly browned.
3. Carefully add the water and liquid aminos, and bring to a boil.
4. Reduce heat to low.
5. Cover and let simmer for 35-40 minutes. Do not stir.
6. Turn off heat and let steam for 15 minutes.
7. Fluff with fork and serve.
8. Flavor with liquid aminos if you'd like.

Servings: 7

Preparation Time: 5 minutes
Cooking Time: 45 minutes
Total Time: 1 hour

Nutrition Facts

Serving size: 1/7 of a recipe (1.6 ounces).

Amount Per Serving	
Calories	198.44
Calories From Fat (3%)	5.58
	% Daily Value
Total Fat 0.63g	<1%
Saturated Fat 0.09g	<1%
Cholesterol 0mg	0%
Sodium 70.68mg	3%
Potassium 48.6mg	1%
Total Carbohydrates 42.98g	14%
Fiber 0.72g	3%
Sugar 0g	
Protein 5.97g	12%
MyPoints 3.88	

Recipe Tips

Massage or personal trainer? If you can't afford both, quit spending money on the massage therapist during your pre-fitness/weight loss goals. Spend the money on a trainer instead. After you better understand your fitness program, your fit foods program, and you have reached your goal and are now in maintenance mode, then go back to getting massages.

* You can cook rice in a rice cooker if you have one. Just hit the brown rice option and let it cook until it shuts off.

Lentils Basic (legume)

Just high protein lentils. 1/4 cup servings. As served at FitBodyRetreat.com.

| 16 | oz | lentils |
| 10 | cups | water |

| 1 | ea | onion, chopped |
| 1 | tbsp | macadamia nut oil (or olive oil) |

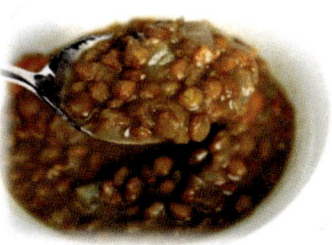

Procedure

1. Bring water to a boil.
2. Add bag of lentils, onion and oil to the pot.
3. Simmer for 45 min.

Servings: 13

Preparation Time: 10 minutes
Cooking Time: 45 minutes
Total Time: 1 hour

Nutrition Facts

Serving size: 1/13 of a recipe (8 ounces).

Amount Per Serving	
Calories	136.16
Calories From Fat (10%)	13.07
	% Daily Value
Total Fat 1.46g	2%
Saturated Fat 0.06g	<1%
Cholesterol 0mg	0%
Sodium 7.94mg	<1%
Potassium 348.77mg	10%
Total Carbohydrates 21.84g	7%
Fiber 10.8g	43%
Sugar 1.11g	
Protein 9.11g	18%
MyPoints 2.04	

Recipe Tips

Some thoughts on bread and beer -- bread and beer will never allow you to reach your fat loss goals! I add them to my cheat day only. If I must use bread for anything, it's only a 35-calorie bread that I will use. If you must drink alcohol, red wine is a better choice than beer. In fact, beer is not even an option during your pre-goal stage of weight loss. And after reaching goal, it's still a forbidden fruit if you want to maintain your new weight.

Lentils with Tomatoes (legume)

A middle eastern dish with a deliciously simple taste. Serve with rice, quinoa and your meat of choice, or whatever you'd like. As served at FitBodyRetreat.com.

1	qt	water
1	cup	lentils, fresh
3	tbsp	extra virgin olive oil
1	ea	green pepper, medium, chopped
1	ea	onion, medium, chopped
2-1/2	cups	tomatoes, peeled, seeded and chopped
1/4	tsp	black pepper
1	squirt	Bragg Liquid Aminos

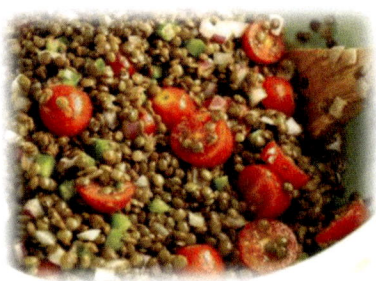

Procedure

1. In a pot, bring the water to a boil.
2. Stir in lentils.
3. Reduce heat and simmer 20 min. Then drain.
4. Heat oil in a large skillet over medium heat.
5. Sauté green pepper and onion until tender.
6. Stir in the tomatoes and season with liquid aminos and black pepper.
7. Add the lentils, reduce heat and simmer for 25-30 min until lentils are tender.

Servings: 4

Preparation Time: 15 minutes
Cooking Time: 1 hour and 15 minutes
Total Time: 1 hour and 30 minutes

Nutrition Facts

Serving size: 1/4 of a recipe (17.6 ounces).

Amount Per Serving	
Calories	299.01
Calories From Fat (32%)	96.34
	% Daily Value
Total Fat 10.96g	17%
Saturated Fat 1.54g	8%
Cholesterol 0mg	0%
Sodium 23.15mg	<1%
Potassium 837.35mg	24%
Total Carbohydrates 37.84g	13%
Fiber 17.16g	69%
Sugar 6.1g	
Protein 14.04g	28%
MyPoints 6.09	

Recipe Tips

Make this up, put it in ½ cup containers; then freeze it, and you'll have a high protein snack in a jiffy.

Quinoa Basic (grain)

This is the off the shelf version. As served at DetoxOasis.net.

- 1 cup quinoa
- 2 cups water
- 1 squirt Bragg Liquid Aminos (or rooster sauce to taste)
- 1/2 tsp macadamia nut oil (or olive oil)

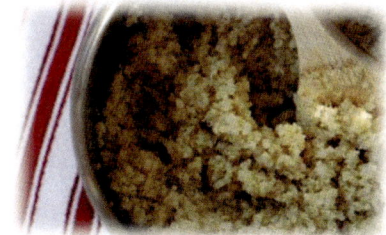

Procedure

1. Rinse quinoa well before cooking. It can be bitter if you don't.
2. Place quinoa, water, liquid aminos and oil into a saucepan and bring to a boil.
3. Simmer 15 min or until tails appear.

Servings: 4

Preparation Time: 5 minutes
Cooking Time: 15 minutes
Total Time: 20 minutes

Nutrition Facts

Serving size: 1/4 of a recipe (6.6 ounces).

Amount Per Serving	
Calories	161.4
Calories From Fat (18%)	28.42
	% Daily Value
Total Fat 3.16g	5%
Saturated Fat 0.3g	2%
Cholesterol 0mg	0%
Sodium 10.68mg	<1%
Potassium 240.46mg	7%
Total Carbohydrates 27.27g	9%
Fiber 2.98g	12%
Sugar 0g	
Protein 6g	12%
MyPoints 2.9	

Recipe Tips

Add any veggies that you wish to or find recipes online. Remember this about quinoa -- it's packed with protein. It's also high in calories. The more ingredients you add to the mix, the higher the calories. I like to use a bit of rooster sauce (or Sriracha) and some Bragg Liquid Aminos for seasoning after it's cooked and on my plate. Bragg has 0 calories and Sriracha has only 1.

A group of "ever so loco" ladies from Toronto, Canada introduced me to quinoa a few years ago -- Anna and Elaine. I had never heard of this grain before that. These gals later came to a Costa Rica retreat with me. Funny how meeting someone and through interaction and discussion, it can influence the foods we eat. These foods then become part of our daily lives. I hope this cookbook becomes a permanent part of your life too.

Quinoa Curry (grain)

A favorite side dish here at the Oasis. As served at DetoxOasis.net.

1-3/4	cups	water
1	cup	quinoa
1/2	tbsp	macadamia nut oil (or olive oil)
1/2	ea	onion, diced (about 4-5 oz)
1	tsp	fresh ginger root, grated
1	tsp	turmeric (heaping tsp)
1	tsp	yellow curry powder (heaping tsp)
1/4	tsp	cinnamon
1/2	cups	frozen peas (or fresh)

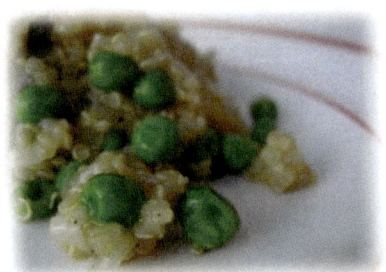

Procedure

1. Add quinoa, water and oil to a saucepan and bring to a boil.
2. Simmer for 20 min.
3. Add remaining ingredients, heat through, and serve.

Servings: 6

Preparation Time: 5 minutes
Cooking Time: 20 minutes
Total Time: 30 minutes

Nutrition Facts

Serving size: 1/6 of a recipe (4.3 ounces).

Amount Per Serving	
Calories	129.86
Calories From Fat (21%)	26.97
	% Daily Value
Total Fat 3.03g	5%
Saturated Fat 0.23g	1%
Cholesterol 0mg	0%
Sodium 16.32mg	<1%
Potassium 208.42mg	6%
Total Carbohydrates 21.23g	7%
Fiber 2.91g	12%
Sugar 1.02g	
Protein 4.78g	10%
MyPoints 2.27	

Recipe Tips

Same ole, same ole, with a spicy twist! Personally, I don't get bored eating the same stuff every day. For me, it's fuel - period. I've included many choices in this cookbook because I don't expect you to like the same foods I do. Treat foods like you do your partner. It's the same ole, same ole routine every day, isn't it? And that seems to work – well, most of the time anyway. Food is the same thing. Mix it up when you must. Stay with what works!

Red Skin Potatoes Roasted (vegetable)

These are great! As served at FitBodyRetreat.com.

- 1 lb red skinned potatoes, washed
- 1 tbsp extra virgin olive oil
- 1 tsp sea salt

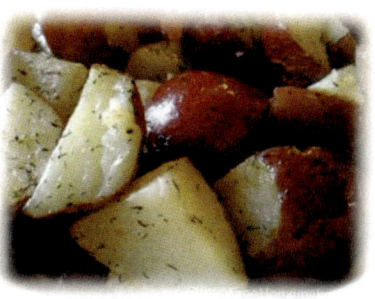

Procedure

1. Rub potatoes with olive oil and sea salt.
2. Wrap them in foil.
3. Bake for 1 hr at 425F.

Servings: 4

Oven Temperature: 425°F

Preparation Time: 5 minutes
Cooking Time: 1 hour
Total Time: 1 hour

Nutrition Facts

Serving size: 1/4 of a recipe (4.2 ounces).

Amount Per Serving	
Calories	119.42
Calories From Fat (26%)	30.61
	% Daily Value
Total Fat 3.48g	5%
Saturated Fat 0.48g	2%
Cholesterol 0mg	0%
Sodium 476.87mg	20%
Potassium 615.8mg	18%
Total Carbohydrates 20.38g	7%
Fiber 1.81g	7%
Sugar 0g	
Protein 2.34g	5%
MyPoints 2.32	

Recipe Tips

These are good, but if you want great, add in a LOT of fresh rosemary!

Rice Pasta - Gluten Free, Wheat Free (grain)

Gluten free, wheat free pasta! As served at FitBodyRetreat.com.

16	oz	Brown rice pasta	1/2 tsp	macadamia nut oil (or olive oil)
1	tbsp	Bragg Liquid Aminos		

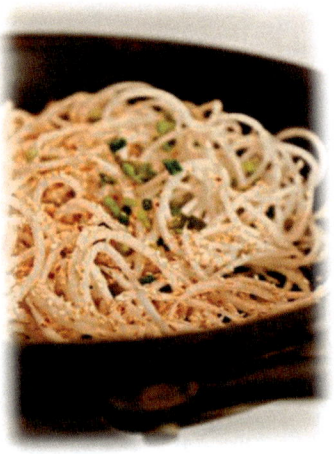

Procedure

1. Boil 4 qts of water.
2. Pour rice, liquid aminos and oil into water.
3. Stir occasionally and cook for 15-16 min until desired tenderness is reached.
4. Rinse with cold water and drain well.*

Servings: 8

Preparation Time: 5 minutes
Cooking Time: 12 minutes
Total Time: 20 minutes

Nutrition Facts

Serving size: 1/8 of a recipe (2.1 ounces).

Amount Per Serving	
Calories	27.5
Calories From Fat (10%)	2.83
	% Daily Value
Total Fat 0.32g	<1%
Sodium 60mg	3%
Total Carbohydrates 5.4g	2%
Protein 0.88g	2%
MyPoints 0.58	

Recipe Tips

Sprinkle with herbs such as parsley or basil if you desire. Here is what I know about rice pasta -- DO NOT OVERCOOK IT, or it will be glue. Follow the suggested recipe, shorten the cook time if you'd like, but never extend it!

* For best results, rid pasta of surface moisture.

Snow Peas (vegetable)

Great flavor and nice crunch when not overcooked.   As served at FitBodyRetreat.com.

? oz   snow peas (amount is up to the chef)

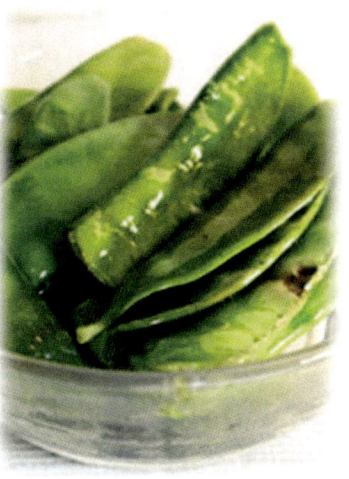

Procedure

1. De-stem and cut ends off of snow peas.
2. Bring water to a boil.
3. Add snow peas.
4. Remove while still firm, about 5 min.

Servings: 1

Preparation Time: 5 minutes
Cooking Time: 5 minutes
Total Time: 10 minutes

Nutrition Facts

Serving size: Entire recipe.

Amount Per Serving	
Calories	12
Calories From Fat (0%)	0
	% Daily Value
Total Fat 0g	0%
Sodium 1mg	<1%
Total Carbohydrates 2g	<1%
Protein 1g	2%
MyPoints 0	

Recipe Tips

Nutritional content is per ounce. Add to any salad, a pile of brown rice, or in any soup. Whether standalone or sprinkled with Bragg Liquid Aminos on top, they're delicious either way.

Spinach, Wilted with Mushrooms (vegetable)

Spinach sautéed with or without mushrooms. This dish creates a perfect base for any piece of meat to sit upon, whether it be fish, chicken or beef. As served at FitBodyRetreat.com.

1 bag (10 oz)	baby spinach	Butter flavored non-stick spray
8 oz	fresh mushrooms	

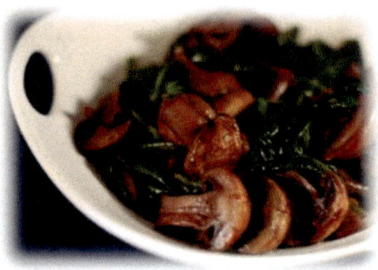

Procedure

1. Heat pan on a medium heat.
2. Spray pan with non-stick spray.
3. Add mushrooms and sauté for about 3 min.
4. Add spinach and sauté with the mushrooms for another 3 min until they appear wilted.
5. Place your favorite meat atop your spinach mushroom mix for an added look and flavor.

Servings: 2

Preparation Time: 5 minutes
Cooking Time: 6 minutes
Total Time: 10 minutes

Nutrition Facts

Serving size: 1/2 of a recipe (9 ounces).

Amount Per Serving	
Calories	57.61
Calories From Fat (11%)	6.57
	% Daily Value
Total Fat 0.94g	1%
Saturated Fat 0.15g	<1%
Cholesterol 0mg	0%
Sodium 117.85mg	5%
Potassium 1152.97mg	33%
Total Carbohydrates 8.85g	3%
Fiber 4.26g	17%
Sugar 2.84g	
Protein 7.57g	15%
MyPoints 0.43	

Recipe Tips

A perfect side or perfect base to set your meat upon for an award winning presentation.

Steamed Broccoli (vegetable)

One of my favorite green veggies - broccoli! As served at FitBodyRetreat.com.

1	bunch	broccoli	1 squirt	Bragg Liquid Aminos (optional)

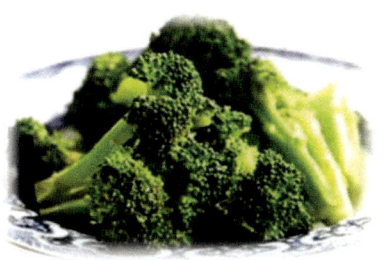

Procedure

1. Heat water to a boil.
2. Break apart the broccoli and add to water.
3. Simmer for 6-8 min.
4. Pull them out while still firm.
5. Season with liquid aminos and serve.

Servings: 4

Preparation Time: 1 minute
Cooking Time: 8 minutes
Total Time: 8 minutes

Nutrition Facts

Serving size: 1/4 of a recipe (1.8 ounces).

Amount Per Serving	
Calories	51.75
Calories From Fat (7%)	3.79
	% Daily Value
Total Fat 0.5g	<1%
Sodium 55.25mg	2%
Total Carbohydrates 10g	3%
Protein 4.25g	9%
MyPoints 1.08	

Recipe Tips

Sprinkle with Dulse flakes or granules if you'd like. Every dinner I eat something green. My favorite selections are broccoli or asparagus – simply based on my taste preference, not on anything else!

Soup & Salad

The Oasis Interior

In your heart of hearts

I go to this place often. What feels right?

I can't stress the importance of this enough. When it comes to food and exercise - although you may not be an expert in these two areas, you still know in your heart if the choices that you make are really the right ones. You know if you eat are eating healthy foods or garbage snacks. And you know if you are exercising enough or not.

Trust yourself, trust your heart, and trust your inner voice. It will be right most of the time. And, if that inner voice doesn't speak to you when you are eating McDonald's or that third bag of chips, then you are going to need additional training! -- and a deeper look into your inner voice.

Talk to a few trainers and get some direction on food and fitness. You will find their advice generally goes along with what your initial gut feeling was telling you in the first place.

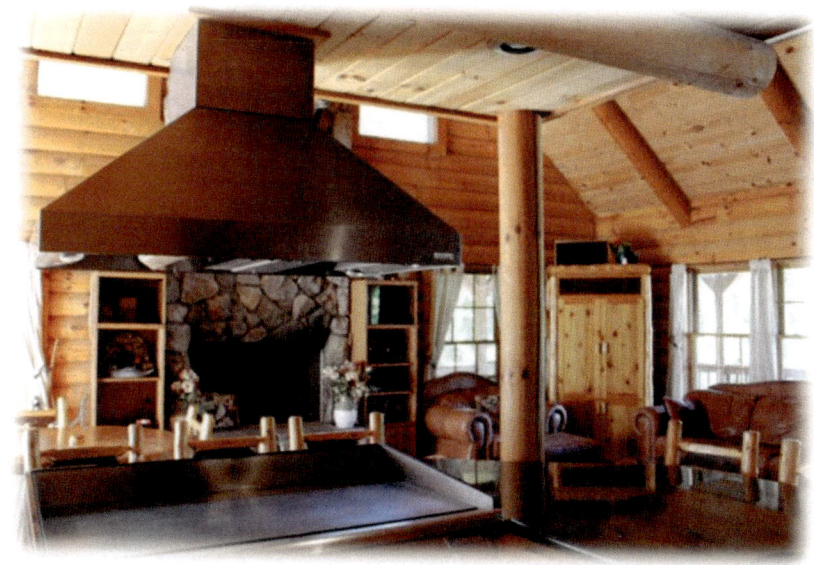

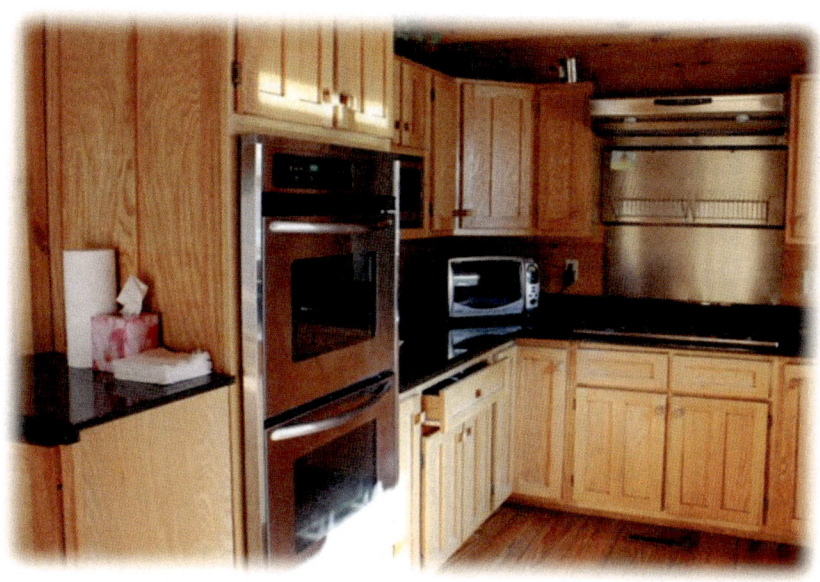

Bean Salad

A spicy bean salad with a kick of lime that is great as a side dish, nacho topping, or all on its own! As served at FitBodyRetreat.com.

14.5	oz	black beans, fresh	1	tsp	cumin
14.5	oz	red kidney beans, fresh	2	tbsp	chili powder
			1	tsp	lime juice
15	oz	garbanzo beans, fresh	4	ea	tomatoes, cubed
14.5	oz	pinto beans, fresh	1	pinch	dried parsley
10	oz	frozen corn, thawed			
1	tbsp	olive oil			

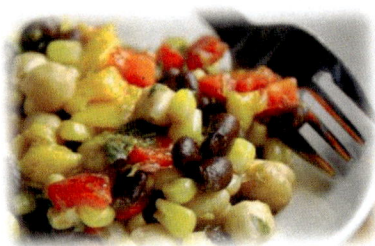

Procedure

1. Cook the beans.
2. Pour beans into a colander and rinse with water.
3. In a large mixing bowl, toss beans and corn together with oil, cumin, chili powder, lime juice and tomato.
4. Sprinkle with parsley, cover and chill.

Servings: 8

Preparation Time: 15 minutes
Cooking Time: 2 minutes
Total Time: 1 hour and 15 minutes

Nutrition Facts

Serving size: 1/8 of a recipe (22.8 ounces).

Amount Per Serving	
Calories	640.98
Calories From Fat (9%)	56.81
	% Daily Value
Total Fat 6.81g	10%
Saturated Fat 0.73g	4%
Cholesterol 0mg	0%
Sodium 51.97mg	2%
Potassium 960.73mg	27%
Total Carbohydrates 130.38g	43%
Fiber 8.99g	36%
Sugar 10.81g	
Protein 27.17g	54%
MyPoints 12.59	

Recipe Tips

Once you hit your fitness and weight loss goals, life is grand! Three meals a day and two protein shakes or bars! Plus, maybe even an extra cheat night is allowed!

Curry Split Pea Soup

This curry split pea soup is terrific! An excellent lunch or dinner. Easy to make and very nutritious. As served at FitBodyRetreat.com.

1	tbsp	macadamia nut oil		1	tsp	curry powder
1	ea	carrot, chopped		4	cups	water
1	ea	onion, small, chopped		1	cup	split peas, yellow or green
1	ea	celery stalk, chopped		1	tbsp	Bragg Liquid Aminos

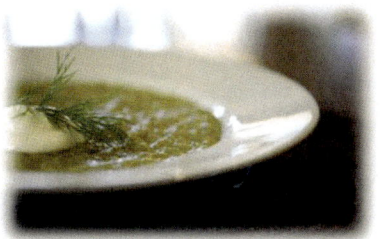

Procedure

1. Heat oil in a large saucepan.
2. Sauté carrot, onion, celery and curry for about 5 min.
3. Add water, peas and liquid aminos.
4. Simmer, stirring occasionally, for about 45-50 min, or until very thick.

Servings: 6

Preparation Time: 10 minutes
Cooking Time: 45 minutes
Total Time: 55 minutes

Nutrition Facts

Serving size: 1/6 of a recipe (8 ounces).

Amount Per Serving	
Calories	143.72
Calories From Fat (17%)	24.2
	% Daily Value
Total Fat 2.82g	4%
Saturated Fat 0.07g	<1%
Cholesterol 0mg	0%
Sodium 105.54mg	4%
Potassium 405.87mg	12%
Total Carbohydrates 22.45g	7%
Fiber 9.15g	37%
Sugar 3.83g	
Protein 8.89g	18%
MyPoints 2.31	

Recipe Tips

I had an Indian guest visit the retreat center, Mahabla from New Jersey. He taught me a few Indian dishes that I make on a regular basis.

Energy Soup

A fantastic cold raw soup to break your detox fast with. We make this soup at the ranch. As served at DetoxOasis.net.

2	cups	water	1	ea	apple, large
2	handfuls	spinach (about 4 cups)	2	tbsp	Bragg Liquid Aminos
1/2	cup	sprouts, small handful (any kind)	3	tbsp	carrots, shaved
1/2	cup	almonds, small handful (soaked overnight)	1/8	cup	blueberries
1	ea	dulse seaweed, small piece	2	ea	pear
1	ea	avocado	1	dash	cayenne pepper

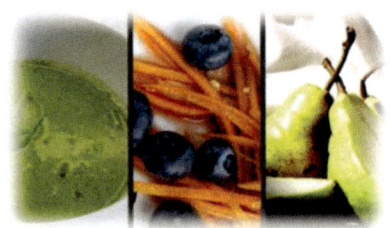

Procedure
1. Set aside a small amount of the carrot, berries and sprouts for a garnish.
2. Add all ingredients except for the pear to a blender. Blend well.
3. Using a large hand grater, grate the pear into a pile.
4. Place the piles of pear into each bowl to create a mountain like appearance.
5. Place the blended cold soup around the mountain of pear.
6. Garnish with a couple of berries and carrots that are cut like a shoe string.
7. Add a few single sprouts.
8. Sprinkle gently with cayenne pepper and serve.

Equipment Needed:
1. Vita-mix or other strong blender

Servings: 6

Preparation Time: 10 minutes
Cooking Time:
Total Time: 10 minutes

Nutrition Facts

Serving size: 1/6 of a recipe (9.6 ounces).

Amount Per Serving	
Calories	180.51
Calories From Fat (47%)	85.38
	% Daily Value
Total Fat 10.57g	16%
Saturated Fat 1.09g	5%
Cholesterol 0mg	0%
Sodium 193.37mg	8%
Potassium 468.74mg	13%
Total Carbohydrates 21.2g	7%
Fiber 6.78g	27%
Sugar 10.81g	
Protein 5.3g	11%
MyPoints 3.69	

Recipe Tips

This is a highly modified version of the Ann Wigmore recipe! If every meal must be an event or a tasty sensation, then you are condemned to a life of misery, sadness and obesity, followed by diabetes and a much shorter lifespan than nature intended for you. Treat food for what it is-- fuel! This dish is really fun fuel! This is the dish we serve our guests on the last day of their detox. It is the first food we serve them as they break their fast.

Ginger Cucumber Salad

A zesty simple plate of cucumbers. As served at FitBodyRetreat.com.

1/3	ea	cucumber, sliced thin		1/2	tsp	oyster sauce
1	tsp	rice wine vinegar		1/4	tsp	hot sauce (Sriracha or rooster sauce)
1	tsp	extra virgin olive oil		1/2	tsp	ground ginger
2	tsp	Bragg Liquid Aminos		1	pinch	sea salt

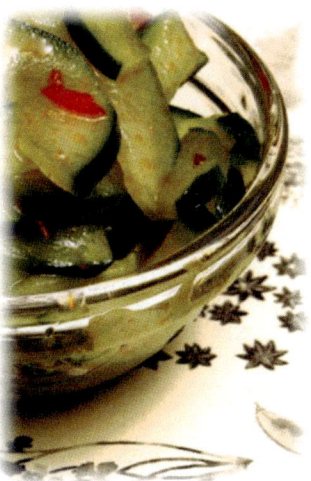

Procedure

1. Slice cucumber thin.
2. Combine remaining ingredients in a bowl except sea salt and mix well.
3. Add cucumbers.
4. Marinate for a few minutes in the refrigerator.
5. Arrange cucumbers nicely on a plate.
6. Add sea salt.

Servings: 1

Preparation Time: 15 minutes
Cooking Time:
Total Time: 30 minutes

Nutrition Facts

Serving size: Entire recipe (4.5 ounces).

Amount Per Serving	
Calories	57.55
Calories From Fat (57%)	32.7
	% Daily Value
Total Fat 4.72g	7%
Saturated Fat 0.66g	3%
Cholesterol 0mg	0%
Sodium 717.8mg	30%
Potassium 191.48mg	5%
Total Carbohydrates 5.33g	2%
Fiber 0.86g	3%
Sugar 1.47g	
Protein 2.74g	5%
MyPoints 1.37	

Recipe Tips

A young lady from Tennessee showed me this dish. It's light, spicy and delicious! Great as a small side or small appetizer.

Ginger Salmon Salad

Ginger salad with amazing flavor! Martha Tejas, a guest here at the ranch, taught me this recipe. As served at FitBodyRetreat.com.

4	ea	garlic cloves	1	tbsp	Bragg Liquid Aminos
1	inch	fresh ginger, shredded	1	ea	Chinese cabbage, small
1/2	dropper	liquid stevia	16	oz	salmon, grilled (4-4oz filets)
1	tsp	extra virgin olive oil			

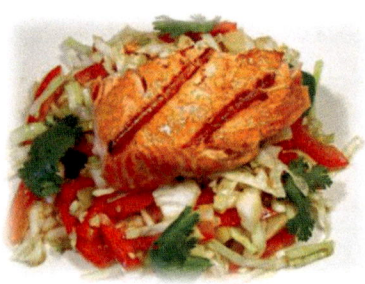

Procedure

1 Pulse garlic and ginger in a food processor.
2 Chop cabbage in a large bowl.
3 Mix stevia, olive oil and liquid aminos together as dressing.
4 Pour dressing over cabbage.
5 Place salmon on top.

Equipment Needed:

1 Food processor

Servings: 4

Preparation Time: 15 minutes
Cooking Time:
Total Time: 15 minutes

Nutrition Facts

Serving size: 1/4 of a recipe (15.9 ounces).

Amount Per Serving	
Calories	235.49
Calories From Fat (38%)	90.47
	% Daily Value
Total Fat 10.2g	16%
Saturated Fat 1.55g	8%
Cholesterol 75.44mg	25%
Sodium 316.61mg	13%
Potassium 1210.57mg	35%
Total Carbohydrates 5.66g	2%
Fiber 2.17g	9%
Sugar 2.52g	
Protein 31.13g	62%
MyPoints 5.13	

Recipe Tips

Calorie management and math. Seriously, how many different ways can I express these thoughts? Wine or dessert? It's got to be one or the other. It can never be both! Personally, I save my calories for a good red wine! Do the math!

Lentil Soup

Hearty lentil soup. Chock-full of veggies and very yummy. Serve with warm cornbread if you like! ~ by Marie

1/4	cup	extra virgin olive oil	2	cups	lentils, fresh	
1	ea	onion	8	cups	water	
2	ea	carrots, diced	14.5	oz	crushed tomatoes, canned	
2	ea	celery stalks, chopped				
2	ea	garlic cloves, minced	1/2	cup	spinach, rinsed and thinly sliced	
1	ea	bay leaf	2	tbsp	vinegar	
1	tsp	dried oregano	1	dash	salt (to taste)	
1	tsp	dried basil	1	dash	black pepper (to taste)	

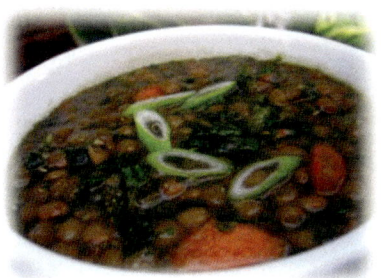

Procedure

1. In a large soup pot, heat oil over medium heat.
2. Add onions, carrots and celery. Cook and stir until onions are tender.
3. Stir in garlic, bay leaf, oregano and basil. Cook for 2 min.
4. Stir in lentils. Then add water and tomatoes.
5. Bring to a boil. Reduce heat and simmer for at least 1 hr.
6. When ready, stir in spinach and cook until it wilts.
7. Stir in vinegar and season to taste with salt and pepper. Add more vinegar if desired.
8. Serve and enjoy!

Servings: 6

Preparation Time: 15 minutes
Cooking Time: 1 hour and 15 minutes
Total Time: 1 hour and 30 minutes

Nutrition Facts

Serving size: 1/6 of a recipe (18.7 ounces).

Amount Per Serving	
Calories	342.81
Calories From Fat (26%)	87.64
	% Daily Value
Total Fat 9.92g	15%
Saturated Fat 1.39g	7%
Cholesterol 0mg	0%
Sodium 193.78mg	8%
Potassium 930.86mg	27%
Total Carbohydrates 47.15g	16%
Fiber 21.83g	87%
Sugar 5.38g	
Protein 17.84g	36%
MyPoints 6.88	

Recipe Tips

Make this up, put it in ½ cup containers; then freeze it. You'll have a high protein snack in a jiffy. We have beans, lentils, wild rice in our freezer made up in advance at all times. They are quick and easy. If I'm hungry -- really hungry, I am prone to cheat if it takes too long to get the fuel. Try to eat every 2-2 ½ hours to stay out of the "I'll eat anything" zone.

Quinoa & Edamame Salad

As served at FitBodyRetreat.com.

1	tbsp	rice wine vinegar		1	cup	cucumber, chopped
1	tsp	macadamia nut oil		1	med	tomato, chopped
1	tsp	sesame oil, toasted		1/2	cup	edamame, shelled, frozen
1	tsp	Bragg Liquid Aminos		1/2	cup	quinoa, cooked*
1/4	tsp	cayenne pepper		1	tsp	sesame seeds

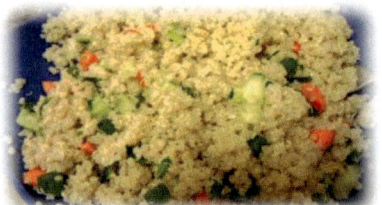

Procedure

1. Cook the edamame according to directions.*
2. Combine rice vinegar, macadamia nut oil, sesame oil, liquid aminos and cayenne pepper in a medium size bowl.
3. Add the cucumber, tomato, edamame, quinoa and sesame seeds.
4. Mix together and serve.

Servings: 1

Preparation Time: 15 minutes
Cooking Time:
Total Time: 30 minutes

Nutrition Facts

Serving size: Entire recipe (16.6 ounces).

Amount Per Serving	
Calories	346.32
Calories From Fat (39%)	136.49
	% Daily Value
Total Fat 17.02g	26%
Saturated Fat 1.4g	7%
Cholesterol 0mg	0%
Sodium 182.08mg	8%
Potassium 1128.37mg	32%
Total Carbohydrates 42.81g	14%
Fiber 9.65g	39%
Sugar 7.13g	
Protein 16.06g	32%
MyPoints 7.54	

Recipe Tips

This is a great dish and satisfying. You're not limited to only edamame when you go for sushi!

* When we make edamame here at our center, we boil it with garlic powder rather than salt.
* See recipe for Quinoa Basic.

Salmon & Cucumber Quinoa Salad

As served at FitBodyRetreat.com.

1	tbsp	rice wine vinegar	1	cup	cucumber, chopped, with skin
1	tsp	macadamia nut oil	2	oz	salmon, cooked
1/2	tsp	sesame oil, toasted	1/2	cup	quinoa, cooked*
1	tsp	Bragg Liquid Aminos	1	tsp	sesame seeds
1/4	tsp	cayenne pepper			

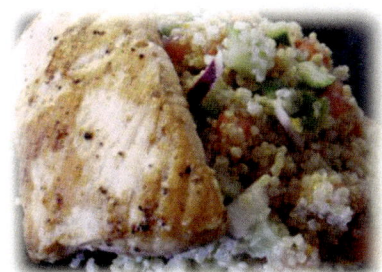

Procedure

1. Combine vinegar, macadamia nut oil, sesame oil, liquid aminos and cayenne pepper in a medium size bowl.
2. Add the cucumber, salmon, quinoa and sesame seeds.
3. Mix well and serve.

Servings: 1

Preparation Time: 10 minutes
Cooking Time: 15 minutes
Total Time: 30 minutes

Nutrition Facts

Serving size: Entire recipe (12.3 ounces).

Amount Per Serving	
Calories	377.73
Calories From Fat (40%)	152.45
	% Daily Value
Total Fat 18.07g	28%
Saturated Fat 1.74g	9%
Cholesterol 66.39mg	22%
Sodium 223.03mg	9%
Potassium 1057.4mg	30%
Total Carbohydrates 29.85g	10%
Fiber 4g	16%
Sugar 1.89g	
Protein 30.23g	60%
MyPoints 8.26	

Recipe Tips

Food is either fuel or fun. Rarely is it both! Treat each meal as fuel, and you will reach your goals much faster. The food fun starts after you reach your body fat and weight goals! Though this dish is pretty good fun for the amount of fuel!

* See recipe for Quinoa Basic.

Spicy Black Bean Soup

Black beans and aromatic vegetables are simmered and seasoned with ground mustard, oregano, thyme and cayenne pepper. Then topped with pico-de-gallo. As served at FitBodyRetreat.com.

16	oz	black beans, fresh, rinsed	2	tbsp	Bragg Liquid Aminos
10	cups	water	1	ea	bay leaf
1	ea	onion, chopped	1/2	tsp	black pepper
2	ea	celery stalks, chopped	1/2	tsp	ground mustard
1	cup	carrots, shredded	1/4	tsp	cayenne pepper
1	tbsp	garlic, minced	1/4	tsp	dried oregano
4	tsp	garlic powder	1/4	tsp	dried thyme
4	tsp	dried parsley			

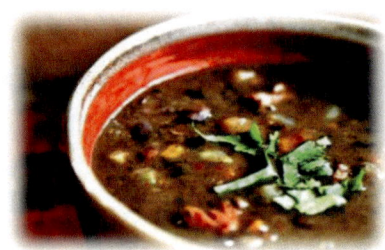

Procedure

1. Add all ingredients to an 8 quart stock pot.
2. Cover and bring to a boil.
3. Reduce heat and simmer for 2 hrs.
4. Discard bay leaf and serve with some pico-de-gallo.*

Servings: 9

Preparation Time: 15 minutes
Cooking Time: 2 hours
Total Time: 2 hours and 30 minutes

Nutrition Facts

Serving size: 1/9 of a recipe (12.6 ounces).

Amount Per Serving	
Calories	86.3
Calories From Fat (1%)	1.06
	% Daily Value
Total Fat 0.12g	<1%
Saturated Fat 0.02g	<1%
Cholesterol 0mg	0%
Sodium 132.97mg	6%
Potassium 116.07mg	3%
Total Carbohydrates 16.79g	6%
Fiber 0.98g	4%
Sugar 1.4g	
Protein 4.92g	10%
MyPoints 1.54	

Recipe Tips

As I keep saying -- make your life easy! Turn this into your "reach for fast food" meal! Freeze it up in 1/2 cup containers. God save me from the raw foodists for suggesting this, but when you need a quick meal, just microwave it for 2 minutes and serve it up!

* Add one cup of rice or quinoa for a perfect meal! Or eat alone as a snack.
* See recipe for Pico-de-Gallo.

Spinach Salad

A simple salad packed with nutrition and protein. As served at FitBodyRetreat.com.

2	handfuls	spinach (about 4 cups)	1	ea	green onion
1	ea	tomato, medium	1/2	ea	red pepper
1/2	ea	cucumber	1	ea	chicken breast (4 oz), cooked or tuna

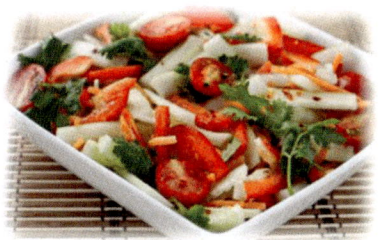

Procedure

1. Mix ingredients together.
2. Top with meat.
3. For a dressing, add equal amounts of Bragg Liquid Aminos and rice vinegar (or apple cider vinegar).

Servings: 1

Preparation Time: 5 minutes
Cooking Time:
Total Time: 5 minutes

Nutrition Facts

Serving size: Entire recipe (20.2 ounces).

Amount Per Serving	
Calories	236.19
Calories From Fat (16%)	37.4
	% Daily Value
Total Fat 4.25g	7%
Saturated Fat 1.01g	5%
Cholesterol 72.29mg	24%
Sodium 172.39mg	7%
Potassium 1586.1mg	45%
Total Carbohydrates 18.01g	6%
Fiber 7.13g	29%
Sugar 9.29g	
Protein 32.82g	66%
MyPoints 4.28	

Recipe Tips

I use whatever leftover meat is in the refrigerator from a previous meal. The spinach comes prewashed from a bag, so it's quick and easy. Remember -- the key to keeping calorie content low with any salad is to be careful with your dressings. If you like this, you will also like the Ceviche recipe.

Spinach, Cabbage & Tuna Salad

As served at FitBodyRetreat.com.

3	oz	tuna, water packed	1	cup	cabbage
2/3	cup	celery, diced	2	tbsp	mayonnaise, light
1/2	ea	tomato, diced	1	ea	bread, low calorie (35 cal. max) and low calorie spread if desired
1/4	cup	chick peas, fresh, cooked			
5	ea	black olives	1/2	cup	grapes
1	cup	spinach (or mixed greens)			

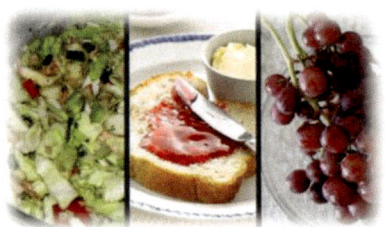

Procedure

1. Mix together in a medium sized bowl the tuna, celery, tomato, chick peas and olives.
2. In a separate bowl, mix spinach and cabbage.
3. Pour 1 tbsp of mayonnaise on top.
4. Place tuna mixture over greens.
5. Drizzle remaining tbsp of mayonnaise over top.
6. Serve a medium sized bunch of grapes and bread with low-calories spread on the side.

Servings: 1

Preparation Time: 10 minutes
Cooking Time:
Total Time: 15 minutes

Nutrition Facts

Serving size: Entire recipe (17.3 ounces).

Amount Per Serving	
Calories	439.34
Calories From Fat (32%)	141.8
	% Daily Value
Total Fat 16.29g	25%
Saturated Fat 2.72g	14%
Cholesterol 46.22mg	15%
Sodium 961.31mg	40%
Potassium 1091.3mg	31%
Total Carbohydrates 47.46g	16%
Fiber 9.1g	36%
Sugar 20.87g	
Protein 29.45g	59%
MyPoints 9.34	

Recipe Tips

Look at the protein content in this recipe! If you weigh 200 pounds, you need 100 grams of protein a day. Remember to get your protein! You will feel fuller and you will build lean muscle!

Spinach, Pepper & Cheese Salad

This is a delicious salad that takes very little time to prepare. As served at FitBodyRetreat.com.

1	pkg (6 oz)	baby spinach	1/4	cup	rice vinegar
1	ea	red pepper, chopped	6	ea	chicken breast, cooked, chopped (small breasts, about 4 oz per breast)
1/4	cup	parmesan cheese			
1/4	cup	Bragg Liquid Aminos*			

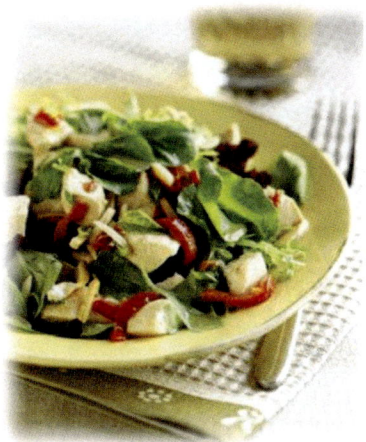

Procedure

1. In a large bowl, mix the baby spinach, red pepper and parmesan cheese.
2. In a small bowl, mix the liquid aminos and rice vinegar for the dressing.
3. Add chopped chicken to salad.
4. Add dressing onto salad and toss.

Servings: 6

Preparation Time: 15 minutes
Cooking Time:
Total Time: 15 minutes

Nutrition Facts

Serving size: 1/6 of a recipe (5.7 ounces).

Amount Per Serving	
Calories	173.71
Calories From Fat (21%)	36.03
	% Daily Value
Total Fat 4.41g	7%
Saturated Fat 1.6g	8%
Cholesterol 75.96mg	25%
Sodium 470.85mg	20%
Potassium 503.59mg	14%
Total Carbohydrates 6.87g	2%
Fiber 1.13g	5%
Sugar 1.17g	
Protein 31.04g	62%
MyPoints 3.62	

Recipe Tips

* You can substitute liquid aminos with same amount of olive oil, but calories go up considerably.

Thai-Green Curry Soup

Hot! "Bring a sweat on Curry Soup that everyone who likes spicy foods will enjoy!" As served at FitBodyRetreat.com.

1	tbsp	extra virgin olive oil		
2	handfuls	chicken (or any meat - about 2 cups)*		
2	tbsp	green curry paste		
2	handfuls	snow peas		
2	can (13.5 oz)	coconut milk, lite*		
1/2	can (15 oz)	chicken stock, lite, low sodium*		
2	ea	kaffir lime leaves		
3	tbsp	fish sauce, low sodium*		
2	tbsp	agave		

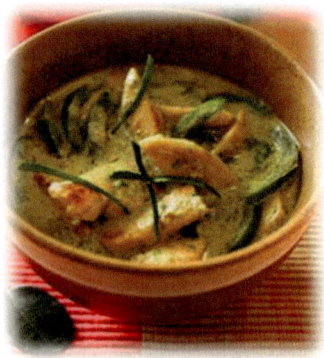

Procedure

1. Place oil, meat and curry paste in a non-stick pan.
2. Cook until meat is about 1/2 done.
3. Add the coconut milk and chicken stock.
4. Add snow peas and remaining ingredients.
5. Bring to a boil.
6. Simmer until the snow peas are done, about 3 min if you want them firm.

Servings: 4

Preparation Time: 10 minutes
Cooking Time: 10 minutes
Total Time: 20 minutes

Nutrition Facts

Serving size: 1/4 of a recipe (19.5 ounces).

Amount Per Serving	
Calories	281.45
Calories From Fat (64%)	181.32
	% Daily Value
Total Fat 16.9g	26%
Saturated Fat 0.87g	4%
Cholesterol 45.36mg	15%
Sodium 1042.69mg	43%
Potassium 262.27mg	7%
Total Carbohydrates 5.48g	2%
Fiber 0g	0%
Sugar 0.75g	
Protein 15.52g	31%
MyPoints 7.04	

Recipe Tips

I learned all the Thai dishes in this cookbook while boxing in Thailand. I make this particular dish more than the others. If you want it to cause a runny nose, just double the green curry. If you want fewer calories, use lite coconut milk. I often make it with salmon and scallops rather than chicken.

* You can use regular coconut milk and chicken stock instead of the lite version in this recipe. However, if you're trying to limit calories, use lite.
* If you want the soup thicker, use less chicken stock.
* You can substitute fish sauce with Bragg Liquid Aminos for a healthier alternative.
* My favorite meats in this soup are salmon cubes, scallops, or shrimp. Chicken is good too.

Thai-Herb Salad

Hot, spicy and yummy! Perfect salad that hits all the flavors. As served at FitBodyRetreat.com.

1	handful	cabbage, savoy (about 2 cup)
1/2	handful	carrots, sliced thin like matchsticks (about 1/2 cup)
1/2	handful	cucumber, peeled and sliced thin like matchsticks (about 1/2 cup)
1/2	ea	tomato, cubed
2	ea	Thai shallots (or any shallots)
1/2	handful	red chili peppers, sliced think like matchsticks (about 1/2 cup)*
1/2	handful	lemon grass, chopped (about 1/2 cup)
1	tbsp	extra virgin olive oil
1	tbsp	Bragg Liquid Aminos
1	tbsp	oyster sauce
1	tbsp	agave
2	tbsp	lemon juice

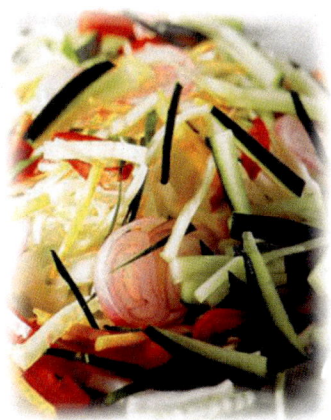

Procedure

1. Mix all together in a bowl.
2. Add lemon juice last.

Servings: 2

Preparation Time: 15 minutes
Cooking Time:
Total Time: 15 minutes

Nutrition Facts

Serving size: 1/2 of a recipe (14.7 ounces).

Amount Per Serving	
Calories	177.46
Calories From Fat (39%)	69.64
	% Daily Value
Total Fat 7.32g	11%
Saturated Fat 1.01g	5%
Cholesterol 0mg	0%
Sodium 548.28mg	23%
Potassium 675.01mg	19%
Total Carbohydrates 20.41g	7%
Fiber 4.27g	17%
Sugar 6.71g	
Protein 5.09g	10%
MyPoints 3.36	

Recipe Tips

I make this at my center every week. It's a spicy favorite. All who try it seem to like it.

* When I can't find a good hot chili pepper, I'll use Sriracha or rooster sauce

Snacks & Dips

The Oasis Lodge

If you are on track with a weight or fat loss goal, then your best choices are always high protein snacks. They not only make you feel full, but they also help you build more lean muscle. And that new lean muscle burns more calories. At night, we suggest you reach for half of a chicken breast, a burger no bun, some tofu or a tasty chocolate protein shake. These choices will build muscle, satisfy your hunger and keep you lean.

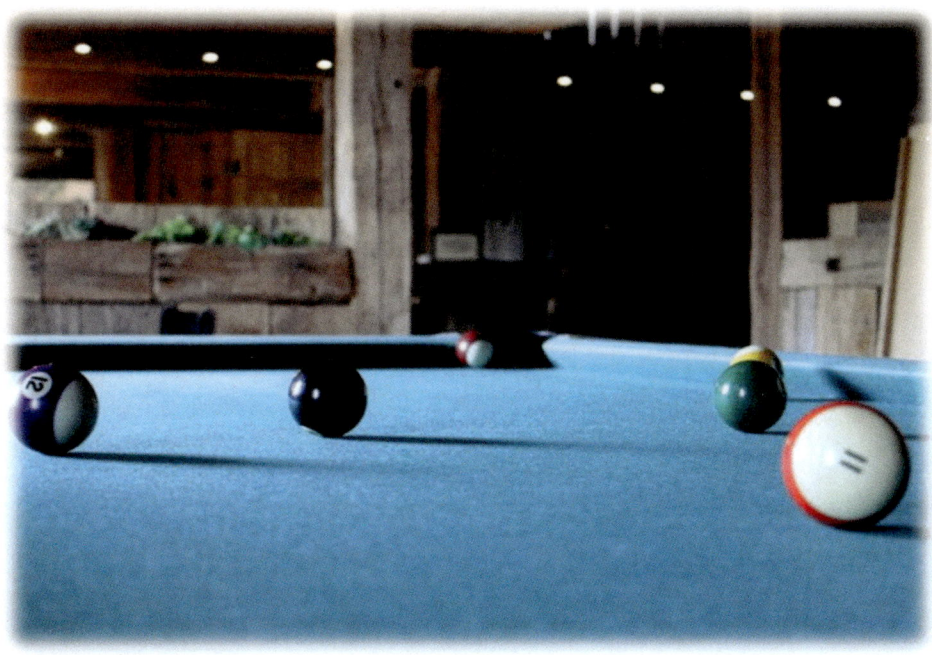

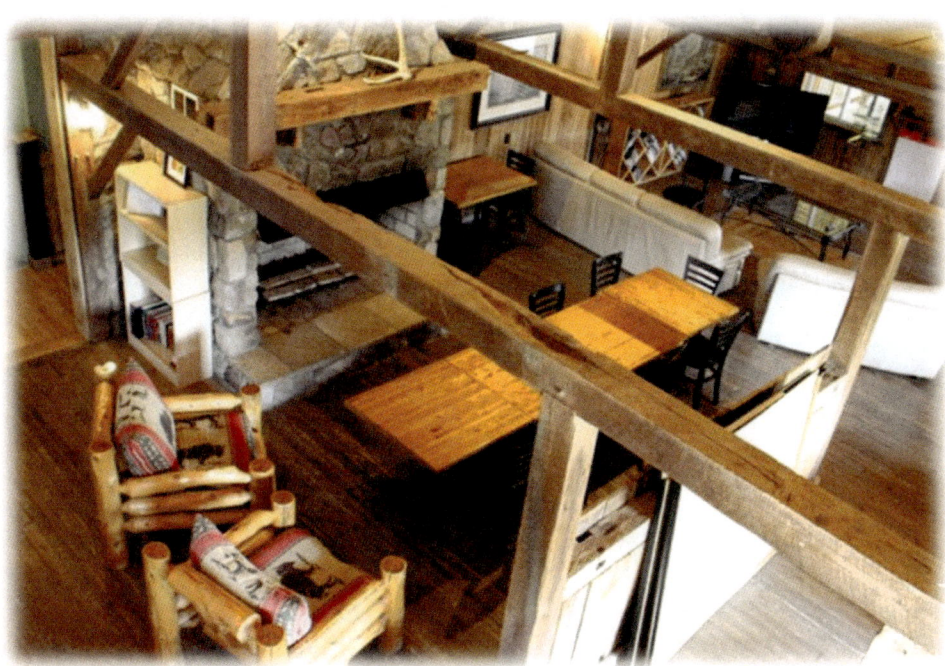

Basil Pesto

This is a pesto we serve fresh from our herb garden. As served at FitBodyRetreat.com.

2	cups	fresh basil		1	tsp	nutritional yeast
1/2	cup	macadamia nut oil		1/2	tsp	sea salt*
3	ea	garlic cloves				
1/2	cup	pine nuts (soaked - or any nut you prefer)				

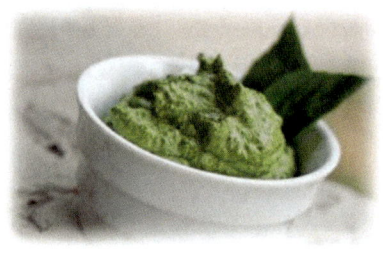

Procedure
1 Put all ingredients in Vita-mix or other blender.
2 Blend and serve.

Equipment Needed:
1 Vita-mix or other strong blender

Servings: 12

Preparation Time: 10 minutes
Cooking Time:
Total Time: 10 minutes

Nutrition Facts

Serving size: 1/12 of a recipe (1.1 ounces).

Amount Per Serving	
Calories	121.37
Calories From Fat (93%)	112.47
	% Daily Value
Total Fat 13.31g	20%
Saturated Fat 0.28g	1%
Cholesterol 0mg	0%
Sodium 79.11mg	3%
Potassium 57.44mg	2%
Total Carbohydrates 1.25g	<1%
Fiber 0.34g	1%
Sugar 0.23g	
Protein 1.12g	2%
MyPoints 3.47	

Recipe Tips

Every summer, I have an herb garden at the ranch. You cannot go wrong with basil, and this recipe is about as raw as you will get. Serve it up with the Mexican Flax Crackers in this cookbook and you will be the pride of the raw food movement!

* Can use Bragg Liquid Aminos as a substitute for salt.
* See recipe for Mexican Flax Crackers

Hard Boiled Eggs & Hummus

As served at FitBodyRetreat.com.

2	ea	eggs, hard boiled	1/4	tsp	paprika
1	tbsp	hummus	1	med	orange

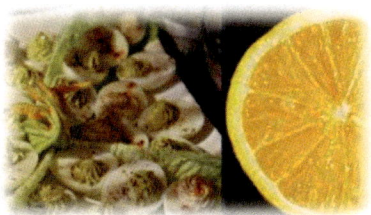

Procedure

1. Cut eggs in half and remove yolks.
2. Mix hummus with one boiled egg yolk. Throw out other yolk.
3. Spoon mixture into hollowed out eggs.
4. Sprinkle with paprika.
5. Serve with an orange.

Servings: 1

Preparation Time: 5 minutes
Cooking Time: 4 minutes
Total Time: 10 minutes

Nutrition Facts

Serving size: Entire recipe (10.2 ounces).

Amount Per Serving	
Calories	304.65
Calories From Fat (40%)	122.65
	% Daily Value
Total Fat 13.91g	21%
Saturated Fat 3.96g	20%
Cholesterol 424.29mg	141%
Sodium 180.92mg	8%
Potassium 494.03mg	14%
Total Carbohydrates 29.25g	10%
Fiber 7.96g	32%
Sugar 1.37g	
Protein 17.19g	34%
MyPoints 6.45	

Recipe Tips

Fantastic snack! These are even better is you don't actually have to make them yourself.

High Protein Chips & Salsa

As served at FitBodyRetreat.com.

1/3	cup	cottage cheese, low fat 1%	10-12	ea	chips, low calorie baked whole grain
4	tbsp	pico-de-gallo*			

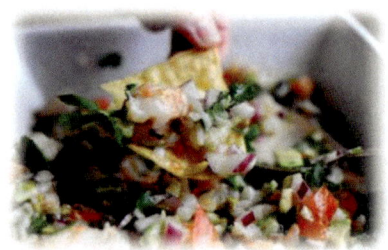

Procedure

1. Mix the pico-de-gallo and cottage cheese together.
2. Serve with low calorie chips or flax crackers*.

Servings: 1

Preparation Time: 1 minute
Cooking Time:
Total Time: 5 minutes

Nutrition Facts

Serving size: Entire recipe (53.2 ounces).

Amount Per Serving	
Calories	165.3
Calories From Fat (19%)	31.16
	% Daily Value
Total Fat 3.4g	5%
Saturated Fat 0.06g	<1%
Cholesterol 0.38mg	<1%
Sodium 528.33mg	22%
Potassium 8.12mg	<1%
Total Carbohydrates 26.26g	9%
Fiber 0g	0%
Sugar 0.26g	
Protein 6.67g	13%
MyPoints 3.59	

Recipe Tips

I really love this dish, especially with elk meat added! But there are a lot of my clients that try to avoid meat as much as possible. This is an alternative to the standard nachos and with a decent amount of protein.

* See recipe for Pico-de-Gallo.
* See recipe for Mexican Flax Crackers if you prefer crackers.

Mexican Flax Crackers

Nice crackers that are all raw, not processed! As served at DetoxOasis.net.

3	cups	flax seeds (soaked 2 hrs)	2	tbsp	chili powder
4	med	tomatoes	2	tsp	cilantro, dried
1	ea	red pepper	1	tsp	garlic powder
1/2	cup	Bragg Liquid Aminos			

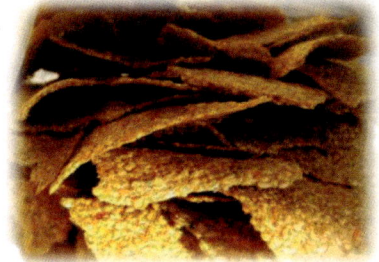

Procedure
1. Soak the flax seeds in 6 cups of water for 4-6 hours.
2. Blend the tomatoes and red pepper in a Vita-mix or other blender.
3. Add the rest of the ingredients to the Vita-mix.
4. Spread the mixture as thin as possible on a teflex sheet - about 1/4" thick.
5. Set in dehydrator at 105 degrees for 5-6 hours.
6. Flip the cracker over and remove teflex sheet.
7. Continue to dehydrate for another 4-5 hours or until completely dry.

Equipment Needed:
1. Vita-mix or other strong blender
2. Dehydrator

Servings: 4

Preparation Time: 30 minutes
Cooking Time: 12 hours
Total Time: 12 hours

Nutrition Facts
Serving size: 1/4 of a recipe (12.8 ounces).

Amount Per Serving	
Calories	619.61
Calories From Fat (62%)	384.66
	% Daily Value
Total Fat 42.21g	65%
Saturated Fat 0.15g	<1%
Cholesterol 0mg	0%
Sodium 1076.33mg	45%
Potassium 488.13mg	14%
Total Carbohydrates 47.53g	16%
Fiber 3.87g	15%
Sugar 5.38g	
Protein 10.48g	21%
MyPoints 15.14	

Recipe Tips
If you keep your hands wet, the mixture seems to spread easier. Generally, when I prepare smoky raw cheese, I also make these crackers to go with the yummy cheese. Make sure you dehydrate these well. If they are soft, they just don't digest well.

Pico-de-Gallo

Here is a nice fresh topping for beans, egg dishes, burritos or quinoa. As served at FitBodyRetreat.com.

1/2	cup	tomatoes, seeded and diced	2	ea	limes, juiced
1/4	cup	red onion, diced	2	tbsp	cilantro (plus extra for garnish)
1	tbsp	jalapenos, diced, seeds removed	2	tbsp	Bragg Liquid Aminos
1	tbsp	garlic, minced	1	pinch	black pepper

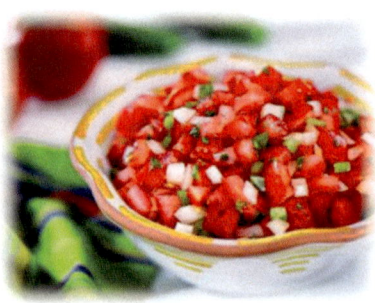

Procedure

1. Mix all in a bowl and place atop your favorite dish or serve with our High Protein Chips or Mexican Flax Crackers.

Servings: 2

Preparation Time: 15 minutes
Cooking Time:
Total Time: 15 minutes

Nutrition Facts

Serving size: 1/2 of a recipe (4.8 ounces).

Amount Per Serving	
Calories	50.48
Calories From Fat (13%)	6.45
	% Daily Value
Total Fat 1.09g	2%
Saturated Fat 0.08g	<1%
Cholesterol 0mg	0%
Sodium 486.51mg	20%
Potassium 254.82mg	7%
Total Carbohydrates 11.93g	4%
Fiber 3.42g	14%
Sugar 2.1g	
Protein 4.81g	10%
MyPoints 0.42	

Recipe Tips

This is great on so many dishes. Great with the Mexican Flax Crackers! Great on omelets! Great with a salad!

*See recipe for Mexican Flax Crackers or High Protein Chips

Protein Bars

8	scoops	protein powder, chocolate	3	tbsp	honey
1	cup	oatmeal (uncooked)	1/2	cup	milk, low fat, organic 1%
1/3	cup	almond butter	3	tbsp	slivered almonds

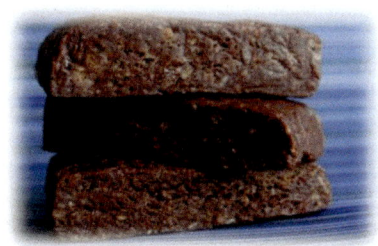

Procedure

1. Mix together the protein powder, oatmeal, almond butter, honey and milk.
2. Form into 4 bars. Then roll into the slivered almonds to finish.
3. Place in refrigerator for about 1 hr.

Servings: 4

Preparation Time: 10 minutes
Cooking Time: 10 hours
Total Time: 1 hour

Nutrition Facts

Serving size: 1/4 of a recipe (5.4 ounces).

Amount Per Serving	
Calories	509.97
Calories From Fat (29%)	149.57
	% Daily Value
Total Fat 16.71g	26%
Saturated Fat 1.32g	7%
Cholesterol 35.52mg	12%
Sodium 154.99mg	6%
Potassium 255.68mg	7%
Total Carbohydrates 49.29g	16%
Fiber 2.88g	12%
Sugar 27.76g	
Protein 41.3g	83%
MyPoints 11.02	

Recipe Tips

These are a bit gooier than the photo above shows. But they are really good!

Raw-Smokey Jalapeno Cheese Alternative

Here is a cheese alternative that's easy to make and has great flavor. As served at DetoxOasis.net.

3	cups	cashews (soaked 2 hrs)	2	ea	jalapeno (remove seeds)
3	capsules	granular type probiotics	1	pinch	onion powder
			1	pinch	garlic powder
2/3	cups	rejuvelac*	1	pinch	sea salt
1/2	ea	lemon, juiced	1/2	tsp	nutritional yeast
1/2	ea	tomato, medium	1	tbsp	liquid smoke
1/2	ea	red pepper			

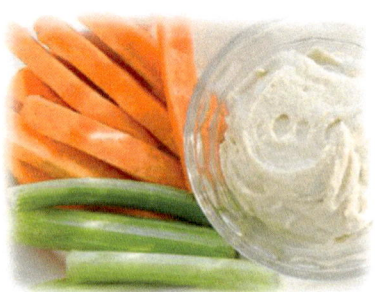

Procedure
1. Mix all ingredients in Vita-mix or other blender until smooth.
2. Line a strainer with a cheesecloth.
3. Set the cheese mixture on to the cheesecloth.
4. Cover the cheese mixture.
5. Store in room temperature for 14-16 hrs.
6. Shape into whatever form you desire.
7. Place in refrigerator for 4 hrs wrapped in plastic.
8. Serve with carrot sticks, celery, or your favorite cracker.

Equipment Needed:
1. Vita-mix or other strong blender

Servings: 20

Preparation Time: 20 minutes
Cooking Time: 20 hours
Total Time: 20 hours

Nutrition Facts
Serving size: 1/20 of a recipe (1.7 ounces).

Amount Per Serving	
Calories	102.37
Calories From Fat (66%)	67.23
	% Daily Value
Total Fat 7.33g	11%
Saturated Fat 0.01g	<1%
Cholesterol 0mg	0%
Sodium 27.01mg	1%
Potassium 18.89mg	<1%
Total Carbohydrates 5.48g	2%
Fiber 0.18g	<1%
Sugar 0.29g	
Protein 3.14g	6%
MyPoints 2.62	

Recipe Tips
Raw foods can be good for you, or they can be just "way too many calories". Listed in this book are a few fun raw dishes to try. You can decide for yourself, based on taste, time to prepare these dishes, and the calorie counts associated with each dish, if they are going to be part of your daily diet. You will love this cheese. I guarantee it! It's fun to make, and your friends won't believe it's raw!

*Rejuvelac is the liquid leftover from soaking wheat grass seeds. You can learn more about making rejuvelac by visiting our Growing Sprouts and Making Rejuvelac recipe.

Raw-Taco's Tasty Meat Alternative

A great raw taco filler. As served at DetoxOasis.net.

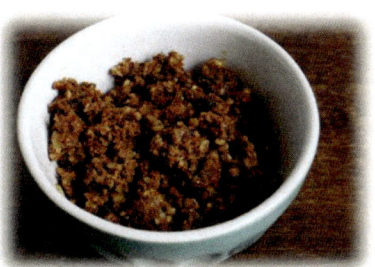

Meat
1-1/2	cups	walnuts, ground
1-1/2	tsp	cumin
2	tsp	taco seasoning
2	tsp	Bragg Liquid Aminos
1/4	tsp	cayenne pepper

Toppings
2	ea	tomatoes
2	tbsp	fresh cilantro
1/2	cup	cheese, low fat (or fat free)
2	handfuls	spinach
1/2	cup	hot sauce*

Wrap
4	ea	Ezekiel 4:9 sprouted grain tortillas

Procedure
1. Pulse the walnuts in a food processor gently until ground.
2. Add remaining meat ingredients and continue to pulse on and off. The idea here is to create a chunky meat like filler. If you pulse too long, it will end up being just a creamy mess.
3. Place cheese on the tortillas and melt in oven.
4. Add remaining toppings. Roll up taco and serve.

Equipment Needed:
1. Food processor

Servings: 4

Preparation Time: 10 minutes
Cooking Time:
Total Time: 10 minutes

Nutrition Facts

Serving size: 1/4 of a recipe (12.6 ounces).

Amount Per Serving	
Calories	419.96
Calories From Fat (50%)	210.51
	% Daily Value
Total Fat 25.05g	39%
Saturated Fat 2.59g	13%
Cholesterol 2.97mg	<1%
Sodium 1222.85mg	51%
Potassium 1183.12mg	34%
Total Carbohydrates 36.24g	12%
Fiber 6.17g	25%
Sugar 2.22g	
Protein 19.84g	40%
MyPoints 9.69	

Recipe Tips

Here is my favorite raw recipe. Simple, fast, and yummy! I serve this dish at least once a week. Erica, from Chicago, taught me this dish. I'll suspect one day she will be a well-known author or advocate. She is a talented writer and chef.

* I like Cholula Hot Sauce!

Veggies & Hummus Dip

As served at FitBodyRetreat.com.

1/2	cup	broccoli tops	5	ea	cherry tomatoes
6	ea	carrot sticks	1/4	cup	hummus

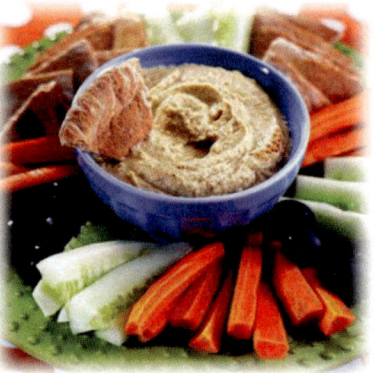

Procedure

1 Arrange vegetables on a plate and serve with hummus as dip.

Servings: 1

Preparation Time: 5 minutes
Cooking Time:
Total Time: 5 minutes

Nutrition Facts

Serving size: Entire recipe (23.8 ounces).

Amount Per Serving	
Calories	335.6
Calories From Fat (17%)	57.72
	% Daily Value
Total Fat 6.82g	10%
Saturated Fat 0.9g	5%
Cholesterol 0mg	0%
Sodium 500.89mg	21%
Potassium 1963.27mg	56%
Total Carbohydrates 64.62g	22%
Fiber 16.95g	68%
Sugar 23.17g	
Protein 9.26g	19%
MyPoints 6.48	

Recipe Tips

This recipe is perfect for any occasion. CONDIMENTS CAN DESTROY A DIET! Let's discuss condiments such as ketchup, mayonnaise, etc. The condiments that people use often add hundreds if not thousands of calories in a week's time. Read the calorie counts and decide if it's really worth it.

Dressings, Sauces & Toppings

The Oasis Gym

It's a known fact, 80% of how we look and feel is how we eat. Only 20% of our look and results is from time spent in the gym!

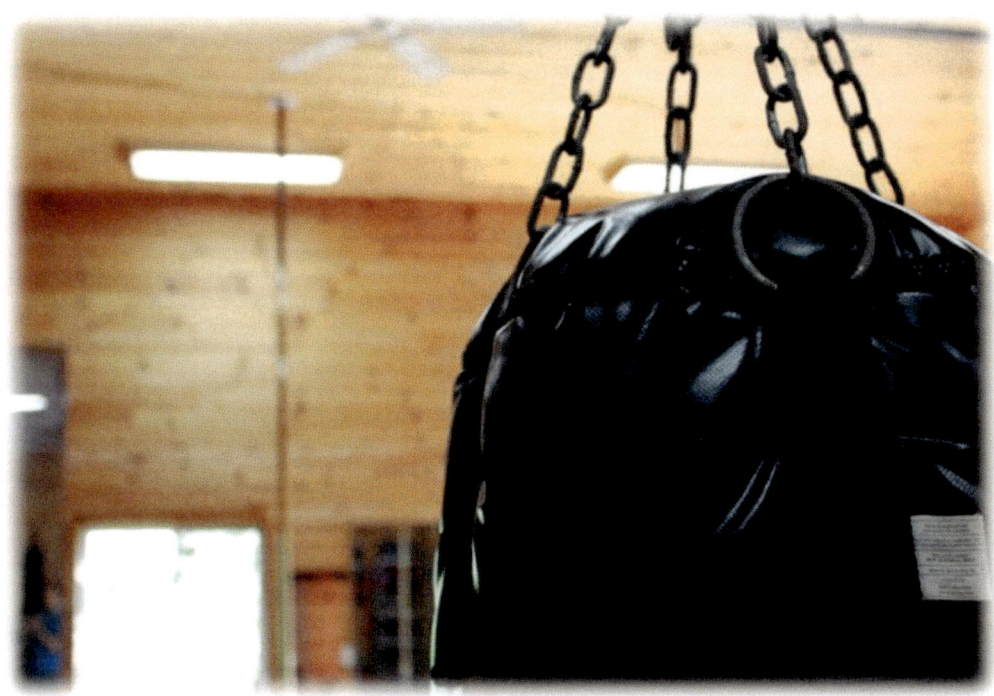

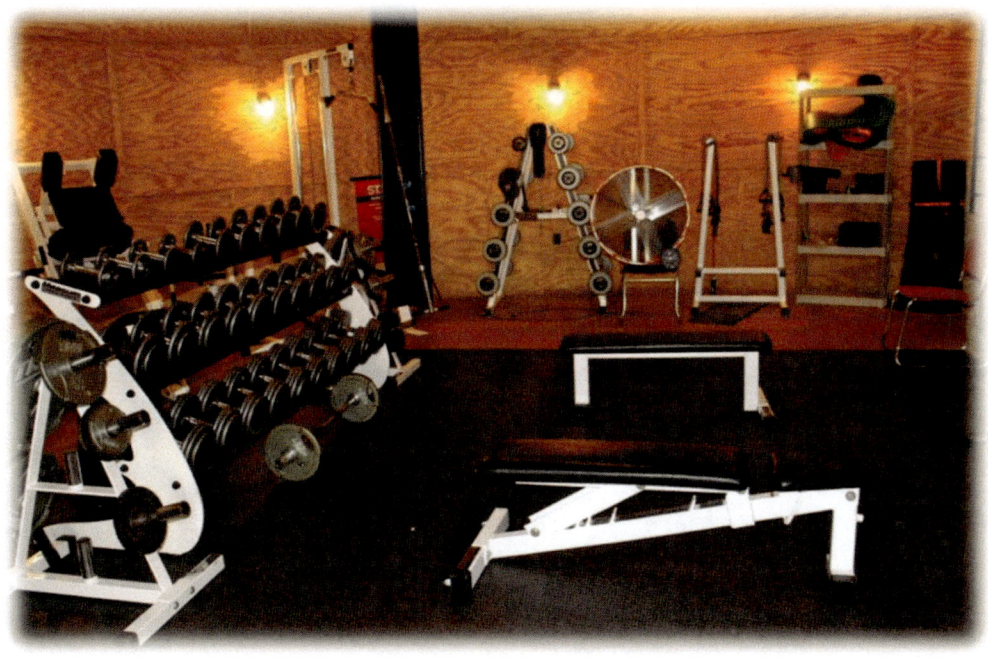

Bearnaise Sauce II

This deliciously creamy herb sauce is so simple to make using a microwave, but if you don't have one, place your bowl over a pan of simmering water to heat it gently. Excellent German recipe for Bearnaise Sauce. Great on steaks, chicken, vegetables and fish. ~ by Chelsea Robertson

1/4	cup	butter	1	tsp	dried tarragon
1	tsp	minced onion	1	tsp	fresh parsley, chopped
1	tbsp	white wine vinegar	1/4	tsp	sea salt
2	ea	egg yolks, beaten	1	pinch	dry mustard
2	tbsp	heavy cream	1	pinch	cayenne pepper
1-1/2	tsp	lemon juice			

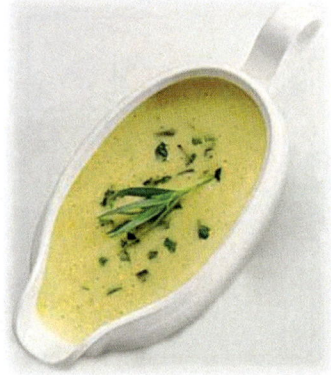

Procedure

1. Place butter in a medium glass bowl and melt in microwave on high for about 30 sec.
2. Whisk together the onion, vinegar, egg yolks, cream and lemon juice.
3. Season with tarragon, parsley, salt, dry mustard and cayenne pepper. Mix well.
4. Return to microwave and cook for 1-1/2 min or until thickened, stirring until smooth every 20-30 sec.

Servings: 1

Preparation Time: 8 minutes
Cooking Time: 2 minutes
Total Time: 10 minutes

Nutrition Facts

Serving size: Entire recipe (5.5 ounces).

Amount Per Serving	
Calories	631.45
Calories From Fat (92%)	583.05
	% Daily Value
Total Fat 66.17g	102%
Saturated Fat 39.27g	196%
Cholesterol 523.33mg	174%
Sodium 617.31mg	26%
Potassium 169.15mg	5%
Total Carbohydrates 5.39g	2%
Fiber 0.39g	2%
Sugar 0.89g	
Protein 6.97g	14%
MyPoints 18.07	

Recipe Tips

I am not a purest! The fact that this recipe is in here is proof! Don't think for a moment I do not put the same garbage in my mouth as most people! I drink my wine when I want to, and I eat the occasional onion rings and pizza. I also love really good micro beers. However, when I'm over my goal weight (meaning outside the 10 pound grace weight that I allow myself), I don't cheat. I dial all of the food rules back to perfect. When you are at your goal weight, you can then splurge on foods like this now and again!

Dave's Favorite Raw Dressing

A creamy delightful dressing that I learned from a raw enthusiast that passed through our doors here. As served at DetoxOasis.net.

3/4	cup	Tahini	1	ea	lemon, juiced
1/4	cup	Bragg Liquid Aminos	1/4	tsp	sea salt
1/2	cup	apple cider vinegar	1/4	cup	parsley
2	ea	scallions	1/2	cup	water
1	ea	garlic clove			

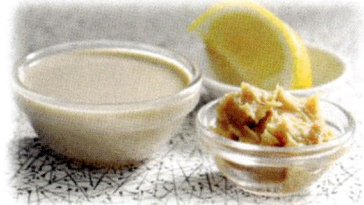

Procedure

1. Add all ingredients to a Vita-mix or other blender and blend well.
2. Serve immediately or refrigerate and serve at a later time.

Equipment Needed:

1. Vita-mix or other strong blender

Servings: 6

Preparation Time: 10 minutes
Cooking Time:
Total Time: 10 minutes

Nutrition Facts

Serving size: 1/6 of a recipe (3.4 ounces).

Amount Per Serving	
Calories	180.72
Calories From Fat (66%)	118.67
	% Daily Value
Total Fat 14.46g	22%
Saturated Fat 2.03g	10%
Cholesterol 0mg	0%
Sodium 424.67mg	18%
Potassium 179.36mg	5%
Total Carbohydrates 9.43g	3%
Fiber 3.05g	12%
Sugar 0.48g	
Protein 7.58g	15%
MyPoints 4.21	

Recipe Tips

One of the nice things about running a center for food and fitness is that you learn a lot of great stuff from others. A raw food chef intern taught me this recipe. It's great!

Pico-de-Gallo

Here is a nice fresh topping for beans, egg dishes, burritos or quinoa. As served at FitBodyRetreat.com.

1/2	cup	tomatoes, seeded and diced	2 ea	limes, juiced
1/4	cup	red onion, diced	2 tbsp	cilantro (plus extra for garnish)
1	tbsp	jalapenos, diced, seeds removed	2 tbsp	Bragg Liquid Aminos
1	tbsp	garlic, minced	1 pinch	black pepper

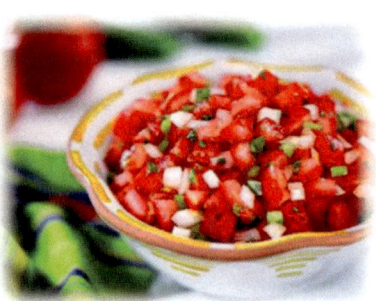

Procedure

1. Mix all in a bowl and place atop your favorite dish or serve with our High Protein Chips or Mexican Flax Crackers.

Servings: 2

Preparation Time: 15 minutes
Cooking Time:
Total Time: 15 minutes

Nutrition Facts

Serving size: 1/2 of a recipe (4.8 ounces).

Amount Per Serving	
Calories	50.48
Calories From Fat (13%)	6.45
	% Daily Value
Total Fat 1.09g	2%
Saturated Fat 0.08g	<1%
Cholesterol 0mg	0%
Sodium 486.51mg	20%
Potassium 254.82mg	7%
Total Carbohydrates 11.93g	4%
Fiber 3.42g	14%
Sugar 2.1g	
Protein 4.81g	10%
MyPoints 0.42	

Recipe Tips

This is great on so many dishes. Great with the Mexican Flax Crackers! Great on omelets! Great with a salad!

*See recipe for Mexican Flax Crackers or High Protein Chips

Raw-Alfredo Sauce

A perfect topping for spaghetti squash or peeled zucchini! As served at DetoxOasis.net.

2	cups	cashews (soaked 2 hrs)	1	tsp	onion powder
1/4	cup	Bragg Liquid Aminos	2/3	cup	water
2	tsp	nutritional yeast	1	pinch	sea salt
1	ea	garlic clove			

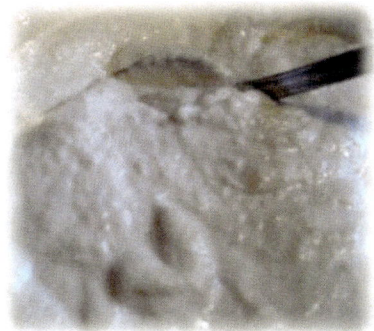

Procedure

1. In a Vita-mix or other blender, add all ingredients and blend until smooth.
2. Serve as desired.

Equipment Needed:

1. Vita-mix or other strong blender

Servings: 4

Preparation Time: 10 minutes
Cooking Time:
Total Time: 10 minutes

Nutrition Facts

Serving size: 1/4 of a recipe (4.2 ounces).

Amount Per Serving	
Calories	86.05
Calories From Fat (56%)	48.56
	% Daily Value
Total Fat 6.73g	10%
Saturated Fat 1.11g	6%
Cholesterol 0mg	0%
Sodium 555.64mg	23%
Potassium 102.87mg	3%
Total Carbohydrates 5.5g	2%
Fiber 0.57g	2%
Sugar 0.89g	
Protein 6.19g	12%
MyPoints 2.17	

Recipe Tips

This is way better than what you will find processed in a jar! Put this on your zucchini slices or your rice pasta. You will love it!

Raw-Ranch Dressing

Wonderful alternative to your typical ranch dressing. 100% raw and tastes great! As served at DetoxOasis.net.

1-1/2	cups	cashews or macadamia nuts (soaked 2 hrs)
3/4	cup	water
3	tbsp	lemon juice
1/3	cup	apple cider vinegar
1/3	cup	extra virgin olive oil
3	tbsp	agave
2	ea	garlic cloves
1	tsp	garlic powder
3	tsp	onion powder
1-1/2	tsp	dill
1	tbsp	sea salt
1/2	tsp	dried basil

Set Aside

1/4	cup	parsley, finely minced
1/2	tsp	dill

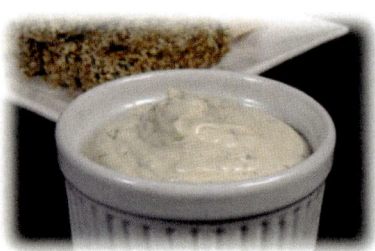

Procedure

1. After soaking nuts, blend all ingredients in a Vita-mix or other blender, except those ingredients set aside.
2. Stir in the set aside ingredients with a large spoon after you are done blending, and serve.

Equipment Needed:

1. Vita-mix or other strong blender

Servings: 8

Preparation Time: 20 minutes
Cooking Time:
Total Time: 20 minutes

Nutrition Facts

Serving size: 1/8 of a recipe (6.5 ounces).

Amount Per Serving	
Calories	232.47
Calories From Fat (74%)	172.75
	% Daily Value
Total Fat 18.05g	28%
Saturated Fat 1.25g	6%
Cholesterol 0mg	0%
Sodium 1181.94mg	49%
Potassium 43.66mg	1%
Total Carbohydrates 7.94g	3%
Fiber 0.33g	1%
Sugar 0.24g	
Protein 6.1g	12%
MyPoints 6.09	

Raw-Sour Cream

This raw sour cream tastes awesome! As served at DetoxOasis.net.

1	cup	cashews (soaked 2 hrs)	1/4	cup	water
1/4	cup	lemon juice			

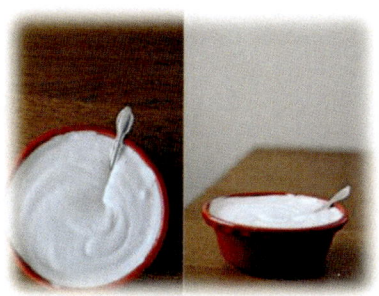

Procedure

1 Add all ingredients to a Vita-mix or other blender.
2 Blend until really creamy.
3 Refrigerate for 2 hrs and then serve.

Equipment Needed:

1 Vita-mix or other strong blender

Servings: 12

Preparation Time: 10 minutes
Cooking Time:
Total Time: 2 hours and 10 minutes

Nutrition Facts

Serving size: 1/12 of a recipe (0.6 ounces).

Amount Per Serving	
Calories	55.45
Calories From Fat (66%)	36.46
	% Daily Value
Total Fat 4.01g	6%
Saturated Fat 0g	0%
Cholesterol 0mg	0%
Sodium 1.2mg	<1%
Potassium 5.29mg	<1%
Total Carbohydrates 3.02g	1%
Fiber 0.02g	<1%
Sugar 0.13g	
Protein 1.68g	3%
MyPoints 1.44	

Recipe Tips

Included in these pages are many raw food recipes. Many of them are fun and healthy. Many of them, in my opinion, are just not worth the calories. I've included the calorie counts for you to make your own decision on what is acceptable to you. Remember to add high fat and high carbs on your cheat day! You must trick that fat storing device of yours!

Spaghetti Sauce

Homemade red sauce that all will enjoy! As served at FitBodyRetreat.com.

2	lbs	ground turkey (may substitute elk or buffalo)
2	tbsp	extra virgin olive oil
1-2	ea	onions, chopped
4-5	ea	garlic cloves
1	can (6 oz)	tomato paste
6	ea	tomatoes, cubed
1	tbsp	Bragg Liquid Aminos (or to taste, add near end of cooking)
1/2	tsp	black pepper
1/2	tsp	onion powder
1/2	tsp	garlic powder
2	tbsp	fresh parsley
1/2	tsp	dried basil (or 2 tbsp fresh, minced)
1/2	tsp	Italian seasoning
1/2	cup	parmesan cheese
1	handful	chopped parsley, fresh (4 tbsp fresh or 4 tsp dried)

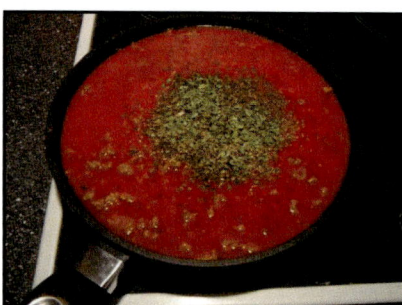

Procedure

1. Cook the ground meat, drain and set aside.
2. Heat oil in a separate pot.
3. Add finely chopped onions.
4. When halfway done, add minced garlic cloves. Cook until browned.
5. Add ground meat to pot.
6. Puree the 6 cubed tomatoes in a blender; then add to pot.
7. Add tomato paste and mix well.
8. Season with liquid aminos, pepper, onion powder, garlic powder, parsley, basil and Italian seasoning.
9. Mix well and simmer for 6 hrs.
10. Top with a pinch of parsley and parmesan cheese.

Equipment Needed:

1. Vita-mix or other strong blender

Servings: 10

Preparation Time: 20 minutes
Cooking Time: 6 hours
Total Time: 7 hours

Nutrition Facts

Serving size: 1/10 of a recipe (7.6 ounces).

Amount Per Serving	
Calories	218.15
Calories From Fat (48%)	105.46
	% Daily Value
Total Fat 11.82g	18%
Saturated Fat 1.29g	6%
Cholesterol 4.4mg	1%
Sodium 350.31mg	15%
Potassium 412.36mg	12%
Total Carbohydrates 8.6g	3%
Fiber 2.07g	8%
Sugar 4.81g	
Protein 19.82g	40%
MyPoints 4.93	

Recipe Tips

Pour this protein packed sauce over anything!

Zero Calorie Dressing

A simple and tasty dressing. As served at FitBodyRetreat.com.

4 tsp Bragg Liquid Aminos   4 tsp rice vinegar

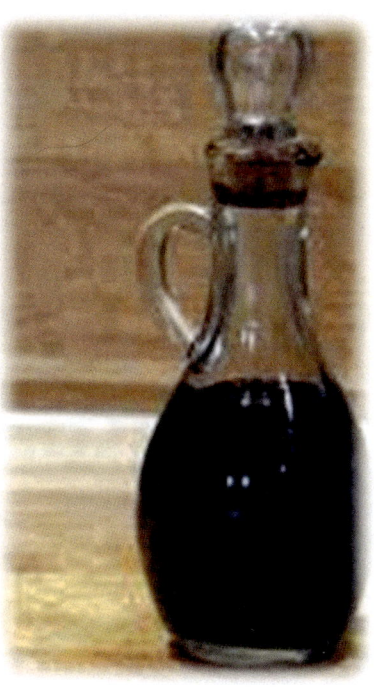

Procedure

1 Mix together and pour on salads.

Servings: 1

Preparation Time: 15 minutes
Cooking Time:
Total Time: 15 minutes

Nutrition Facts

Serving size: Entire recipe (1.4 ounces).

Amount Per Serving	
Calories	2.8
Calories From Fat (0%)	0
	% Daily Value
Total Fat 0g	0%
Sodium 641.43mg	27%
Potassium 142.8mg	4%
Total Carbohydrates 8.42g	3%
Protein 4g	8%
MyPoints 0.06	

Recipe Tips

This stuff is the best! I had an intern from Australia, who stayed at our center for 3 months, teach me this salad dressing. ZERO calories – well, almost zero. Thanks Jules! I use this every day. Caution -- way too many people will make a wonderful salad and then destroy it with 500 calories of processed blue cheese dressing. Use this stuff and your salad will get none of the extra poison or calories associated with the processed dressings that you find at the store.

Dessert

The Oasis Team

The Oasis is a small family managed business on a 120 acre elk ranch in the rolling hills of southern Indiana. We raise our own animals for clean grass fed meats. We grow our own herbs and vegetables in our garden. And we purchase organic foods at the local farmer's markets.

At the Oasis, we run about 20 retreats a year. Most of them are at our ranch in Indiana with a couple of them in Costa Rica. Our retreats typically run 6 to 10 days with the occasional 30 day retreat. We have about 5 to 12 guests with us on any given week.

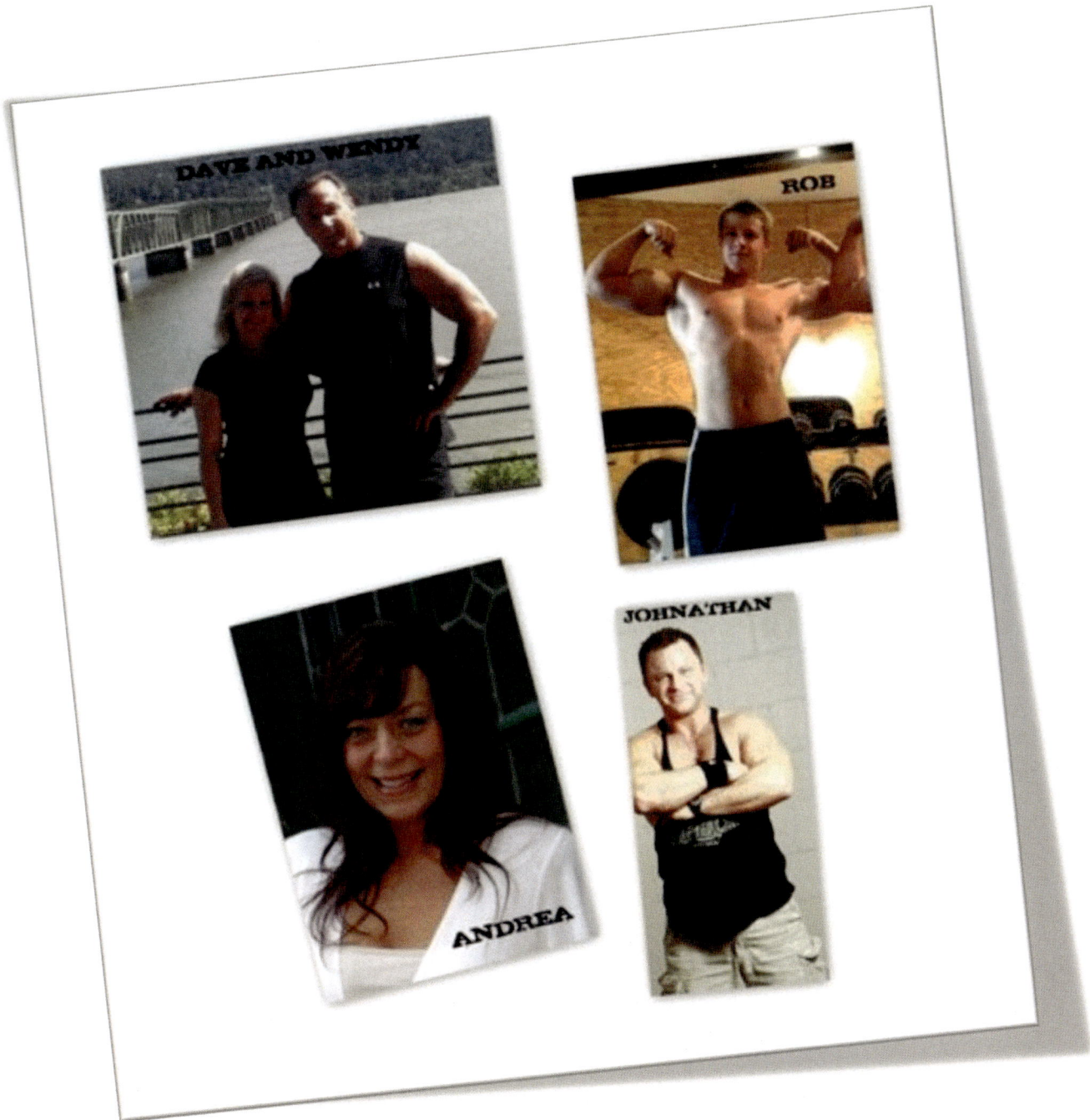

Berries & Yogurt

This is so good! Perfect for that morning when you are not really hungry but know you should eat something good just to get some energy. Your choice of berries - or a combination of them. Strawberries, raspberries, or blueberries. Sprinkled with shaved almonds. As served at FitBodyRetreat.com.

1	cup	vanilla yogurt, fat free
1/2	cup	blueberries, fresh (any berry)*
4	tbsp	almonds, raw shaved

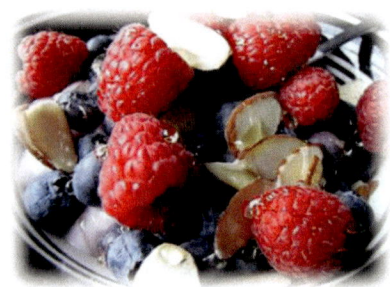

Procedure

1. Pour berries on top of the yogurt.
2. Top with shaved almonds.

Servings: 1

Preparation Time: 5 minutes
Cooking Time:
Total Time: 5 minutes

Nutrition Facts

Serving size: Entire recipe (7.1 ounces).

Amount Per Serving	
Calories	382.13
Calories From Fat (31%)	119.67
	% Daily Value
Total Fat 14.24g	22%
Saturated Fat 0.02g	<1%
Cholesterol 0mg	0%
Sodium 140.74mg	6%
Potassium 56.98mg	2%
Total Carbohydrates 53.72g	18%
Fiber 1.78g	7%
Sugar 7.37g	
Protein 16.55g	33%
MyPoints 8.47	

Recipe Tips

Children can be picky eaters. That is a fact of life. Compensating by feeding them crap because they won't eat the healthy foods you offer them should be a crime that parents need to be held accountable for. When I see a 12 year old 50 pounds overweight, I wonder how a parent could do this to the child they love? Don't they know that diabetes is just around the corner and a lifetime of obesity is their future? If you are a parent, take charge. Do the right thing for your children and give them the best shot at life and health. It's really up to you.

* Calories are pretty close for all the berries.

Cinnamon Apple & Almond Ricotta

As served at FitBodyRetreat.com.

1	ea	apple, medium, seedless	1/4 cup	ricotta cheese, light
5	ea	almonds, raw, unsalted	1/4 tsp	cinnamon

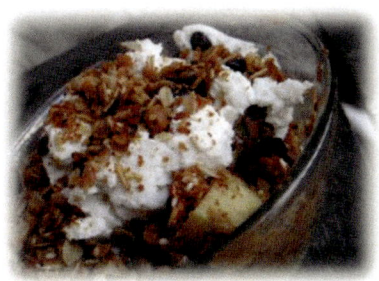

Procedure

1. Cut up the apple.
2. Mix together apple, almonds and ricotta cheese.
3. Top with cinnamon.

Servings: 1

Preparation Time: 5 minutes
Cooking Time:
Total Time: 5 minutes

Nutrition Facts

Serving size: Entire recipe (24.8 ounces).

Amount Per Serving	
Calories	215.62
Calories From Fat (32%)	69.08
	% Daily Value
Total Fat 8.15g	13%
Saturated Fat 3.31g	17%
Cholesterol 19.07mg	6%
Sodium 92.43mg	4%
Potassium 321.25mg	9%
Total Carbohydrates 30.12g	10%
Fiber 5.45g	22%
Sugar 19.35g	
Protein 8.78g	18%
MyPoints 4.19	

Recipe Tips

Yes, it's good! Yes, it's got heaps of sugar and calories! But it's worth a try and it's raw! Remember this though -- just because it's raw doesn't mean that rules do not apply to the dish. Calories are calories!

Coconut Rice & Mango

Yummy side dish! Tastes like dessert. As served at FitBodyRetreat.com.

1/2	ea	mango	1	tsp	Bragg Liquid Aminos	
4	tsp	coconut milk, lite	1	handful	wild rice, cooked (about 1/2 cup)	
2	tsp	agave	1	pinch	cinnamon	

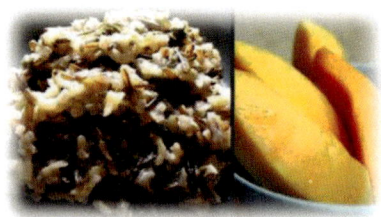

Procedure

1 Peel and slice mango.
2 Arrange sliced mango nicely on a small plate.
3 Pour coconut milk, agave and liquid aminos into a non-stick pan and cook over a low heat.
4 Mix together until well blended, stirring continually.
5 Remove from heat and mix in a bowl with the rice.
6 Form into a ball and serve next to the fruit on the same plate.

Servings: 1

Preparation Time: 10 minutes
Cooking Time: 5 minutes
Total Time: 15 minutes

Nutrition Facts

Serving size: Entire recipe (27.9 ounces).

Amount Per Serving	
Calories	197.62
Calories From Fat (4%)	7.58
	% Daily Value
Total Fat 0.68g	1%
Saturated Fat 0.14g	<1%
Cholesterol 0mg	0%
Sodium 181.52mg	8%
Potassium 257.92mg	7%
Total Carbohydrates 33.23g	11%
Fiber 3.28g	13%
Sugar 14.74g	
Protein 5.13g	10%
MyPoints 3.35	

Recipe Tips

I love this dish. Even more so if someone makes it for me and serves it up! And washes the dishes too? – now I'm in heaven!

Fresh Mango Yogurt

As served at FitBodyRetreat.com.

1/2	cup	plain yogurt, 1%	1/2 cup	mango, fresh, diced
1	tbsp	protein powder, vanilla		

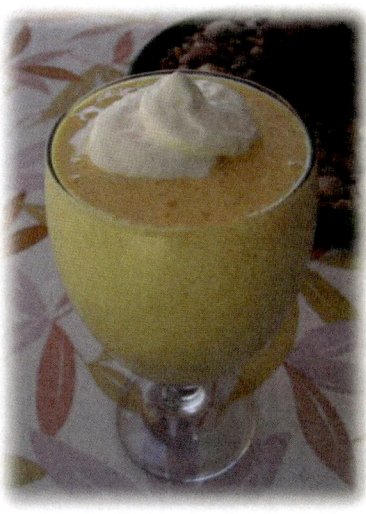

Procedure

1 Mix all ingredients together and stir.

Servings: 1

Preparation Time: 5 minutes
Cooking Time:
Total Time: 5 minutes

Nutrition Facts

Serving size: Entire recipe (10.8 ounces).

Amount Per Serving	
Calories	163.68
Calories From Fat (15%)	23.97
	% Daily Value
Total Fat 3.21g	5%
Saturated Fat 1.3g	7%
Cholesterol 7.35mg	2%
Sodium 229.58mg	10%
Potassium 425.25mg	12%
Total Carbohydrates 28.98g	10%
Fiber 1.32g	5%
Sugar 19.89g	
Protein 13.11g	26%
MyPoints 3.28	

Recipe Tips

By now, I hope you are following the trend here! It's all about high protein and resistance training. Eat high protein and you will feel much fuller than meals loaded with carbs. Eat high protein and include resistance training and you'll add lean muscle. Add lean muscle and you will naturally burn more calories! Add lean muscle and you will look very sexy!

Raw-Apple Sauce

A good sweet dessert that's fresh and 100% raw. As served at DetoxOasis.net.

- 2 ea apples, large (any sweet variety)
- 2 ea dates (any sweet variety like Medjool)
- 1/2 tsp cinnamon

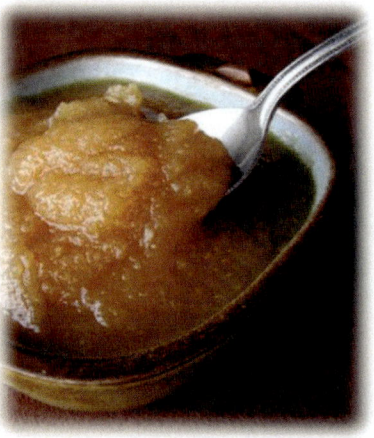

Procedure

1. Cut up the apples into smaller chunks.
2. Place apples, dates and cinnamon in a food processor using the "S" blade.
3. Pulse until chunky but well mixed.

Equipment Needed:

1. Food processor

Servings: 2

Preparation Time: 10 minutes
Cooking Time:
Total Time: 10 minutes

Nutrition Facts

Serving size: 1/2 of a recipe (11.4 ounces).

Amount Per Serving	
Calories	178.57
Calories From Fat (2%)	3.08
	% Daily Value
Total Fat 0.39g	<1%
Saturated Fat 0.06g	<1%
Cholesterol 0mg	0%
Sodium 2.3mg	<1%
Potassium 241.41mg	7%
Total Carbohydrates 49.32g	16%
Fiber 5.7g	23%
Sugar 23.18g	
Protein 0.61g	1%
MyPoints 2.8	

Recipe Tips

Somehow, when I eat this, it just feels "right". How much easier and more natural can it get! Don't forget --calories are calories, raw or not. Make sure you know your numbers and never try to justify high calorie foods by saying "at least it's healthy".

Raw-Berry Cheesecake

100% raw dessert. A delicious cheesecake alternative! As served at DetoxOasis.net.

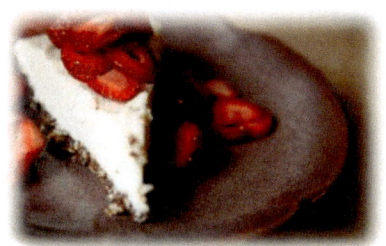

Crust
- 1-1/2 cup almonds (soaked overnight)
- 1 cup raisins

Filling
- 3 cup cashews (soaked 2 hrs)
- 1 cup lemon juice
- 1 cup honey
- 1 cup extra virgin coconut oil
- 1 tsp almond extract

Topping
- 1 bag frozen strawberries (or any other berries, 16-20 oz bag)
- 1/4 cup agave

Procedure

Crust
1. Mix the raisins and almonds in the food processor until fine.
2. Press this mixture into a pie plate.
3. Place in refrigerator.

Filling
1. Blend cashews, lemon juice, honey, coconut oil and almond extract in a Vita-mix or other strong blender.
2. Pour this mixture onto the crust.
3. Put the pie back into the refrigerator for 2+ hrs.
4. Serve after chilled.

Topping
1. Blend the frozen berries and agave in the Vita-mix blender.
2. Pour the topping onto each piece of pie as it is served.
3. Keep topping separate from whole pie and in refrigerator until served.

Equipment Needed:
1. Vita-mix or other strong blender
2. Food processor

Servings: 8

Preparation Time: 30 minutes
Cooking Time:
Total Time: 2 hours and 30 minutes

Nutrition Facts

Serving size: 1/8 of a recipe (8.3 ounces).

Amount Per Serving	
Calories	883.48
Calories From Fat (58%)	509.44
	% Daily Value
Total Fat 58.94g	91%
Saturated Fat 0.03g	<1%
Cholesterol 0mg	0%
Sodium 10.88mg	<1%
Potassium 312.83mg	9%
Total Carbohydrates 83.07g	28%
Fiber 2.43g	10%
Sugar 51.01g	
Protein 14.3g	29%
MyPoints 22.1	

Recipe Tips

You won't find many dessert recipes in my cookbook. Why? Because with me, it's either dessert or wine after dinner. You must choose one! It can never be both. "Please pass the Shiraz!" Note: This cheesecake is crazy good!

Raw-Chocolate Avocado Mousse

Creamy, rich, and completely raw. Your guests will be shocked when they learn it's a raw dessert!

- 4 ea   avocados, ripe
- 1 cup agave (or evaporated cane juice)
- 1 tbsp vanilla extract
- 1 cup cocoa powder, organic fair trade (or carob)

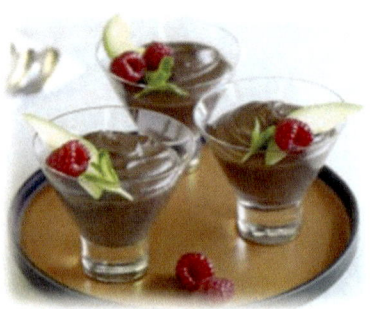

Procedure

1. Slice each avocado open and scoop out the insides.
2. Place the avocado meat in a food processor or blender.
3. Add the agave, vanilla and cocoa powder.
4. Blend or process the mixture until fully blended.
5. Mixture should be smooth and the color of chocolate.
6. Can be served instantly, but tastes better after being refrigerated for at least 1 hr.
7. Serve in small cups with fresh fruit* or a sprig of mint on top - like a peppermint piece you find in some ice cream.

Equipment Needed:

1. Vita-mix or other strong blender, or a food processor

Servings: 4

Preparation Time: 10 minutes
Cooking Time:
Total Time: 1 hour and 15 minutes

Nutrition Facts

Serving size: 1/4 of a recipe (8.8 ounces).

Amount Per Serving	
Calories	559.98
Calories From Fat (45%)	253.44
	% Daily Value
Total Fat 32.41g	50%
Saturated Fat 6.01g	30%
Cholesterol 0mg	0%
Sodium 18.88mg	<1%
Potassium 1307.32mg	37%
Total Carbohydrates 78g	26%
Fiber 20.61g	82%
Sugar 2.11g	
Protein 8.24g	16%
MyPoints 13.1	

Recipe Tips

I was taught this dessert by a good friend, Kat from Bloomington, Indiana. She is working on a project called Spirit Tree Farms. She is into all sorts of funky stuff. This tastes great! But I have to say "no thank you my dear, I'm saving my calories for the wine!" It's a reality and a shame. Unfortunately, it's got to be one or the other after the age of 40.

*Good fruits to top this with are strawberries, raspberries, blueberries, and sometimes pineapple.

Raw-Ice Cream Sundae

What can I say? It's ice cream. As served at DetoxOasis.net.

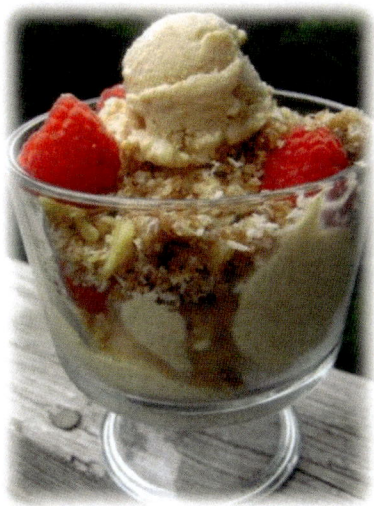

The Base
| 2 | ea | frozen bananas |

The Sauce
2	tbsp	agave
1-1/2	tsp	cocoa powder
1	dash	almond extract

The Toppings
1	ea	dates
1	tbsp	walnuts finely chopped (or any nut)
1/4	cup	fresh raspberries (optional, or any fruit)

Procedure
1. Blend bananas in Vita-mix or other blender until smooth.
2. Mix agave, cocoa and almond extract in a separate bowl and pour over the banana puree.
3. Add the toppings and serve.

Equipment Needed:
1. Vita-mix or other strong blender

Servings: 2

Preparation Time: 10 minutes
Cooking Time:
Total Time: 10 minutes

Nutrition Facts
Serving size: 1/2 of a recipe (16.8 ounces).

Amount Per Serving		
Calories		218.95
Calories From Fat (66%)		145.54
		% Daily Value
Total Fat 42.12g		65%
Saturated Fat 0.56g		3%
Cholesterol 0mg		0%
Sodium 29.16mg		1%
Potassium 128.69mg		4%
Total Carbohydrates 34.81g		12%
Fiber 2.93g		12%
Sugar 3.48g		
Protein 3.15g		6%
MyPoints 7.3		

Recipe Tips
Raw foods are interesting, and most often, very healthy and nutritious. Even more interesting is the cult-like following the raw food movement seems to have!

Raw-Oatmeal Cookies

2 cups oat groats, whole
1/2 cup almonds
1/2 cup raisins
1/2 cup agave (or maple syrup)
1/4 cup cashews

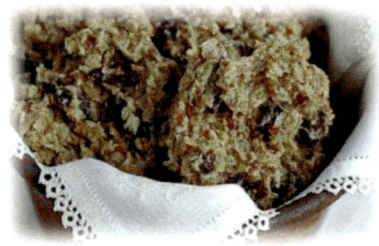

Procedure

1. Put oats in food processor and grind until fine.
2. Transfer to a mixing bowl.
3. Put almonds in food processor and pulse a few times to chop them until just coarsely chopped.
4. Transfer to bowl with the groats.
5. Add raisins and agave to bowl and mix everything well.
6. Grind cashews in a coffee grinder.
7. Use this to coat your palms as you handle the cookie dough.
8. Take small chunks of dough and flatten into round cookie shapes onto the mesh sheet of a dehydrator tray.
9. Dehydrate for about 12 hrs on 110 degrees. Dehydrating time will vary depending on how thick you've made your cookies and the desired chewy/crunchiness.

Equipment Needed:

1. Food processor
2. Coffee Grinder
3. Dehydrator

Servings: 6

Preparation Time: 20 minutes
Cooking Time: 24 hours
Total Time: 24 hours

Nutrition Facts

Serving size: 1/6 of a recipe (3.3 ounces).

Amount Per Serving	
Calories	374.82
Calories From Fat (21%)	77.06
	% Daily Value
Total Fat 9.43g	15%
Saturated Fat 0.78g	4%
Cholesterol 0mg	0%
Sodium 8.15mg	<1%
Potassium 361.93mg	10%
Total Carbohydrates 71.78g	24%
Fiber 7.59g	30%
Sugar 8.6g	
Protein 10.2g	20%
MyPoints 7.48	

Recipe Tips

You can add a couple scoops of chocolate protein powder to this for high protein raw cookies. Be careful though! It's hard to eat just a couple!

Spicy Fruity Thai Sensation

A delicious, fruity, sweet, sour, hot dish that was created here at the ranch using proven Thai cooking principles. As served at FitBodyRetreat.com.

2	tbsp	oyster sauce	1	ea	pear
1	tbsp	Bragg Liquid Aminos	1	ea	avocado
1	tbsp	hot sauce (Sriracha or rooster sauce)	1	ea	mango
4	tbsp	agave	1	ea	lemon, juiced

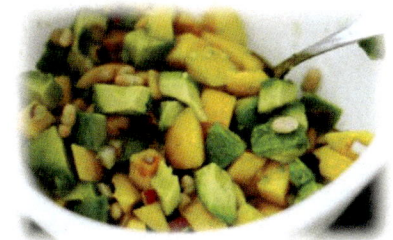

Procedure

1. Cut up fruit into small squares.
2. Combine all ingredients into a bowl or container with lid.
3. Squeeze the juice from 1 lemon onto it.
4. Shake or stir all together. (I prefer to shake)
5. Serve in a small cocktail dish.

Servings: 6

Preparation Time: 10 minutes
Cooking Time:
Total Time: 10 minutes

Nutrition Facts

Serving size: 1/6 of a recipe (11.1 ounces).

Amount Per Serving	
Calories	131.55
Calories From Fat (41%)	53.68
	% Daily Value
Total Fat 4.66g	7%
Saturated Fat 0.65g	3%
Cholesterol 0mg	0%
Sodium 327.14mg	14%
Potassium 256.22mg	7%
Total Carbohydrates 13.62g	5%
Fiber 3.49g	14%
Sugar 7.98g	
Protein 1.59g	3%
MyPoints 2.32	

Recipe Tips

See why wine is good for you? I created this delicious recipe after being over-served on some red wine one night with clients at the Oasis! You will love it. Sweet, sour, hot, and spicy!

Meal Replacements

Oasis Accommodations

Meal replacements are without a doubt the fastest way to assist a person in building lean muscle, losing weight, losing body fat and reaching fitness goals. At the Oasis, we transition into meal replacement shakes the week following a client's detox. It is in the second week of the client's stay that the cooking classes begin and the lifelong knowledge of what to eat and when to eat all comes together and starts to make sense. By the end of the second week at the Oasis, our clients will return home with all of the skills and knowledge they need to either maintain a healthy weight or continue losing five to seven pounds a week on their own.

The Oasis is so much more than just a detox center. Here you will learn lifelong skills in foods and fitness which will enable you to start a brand new life as a fit lean person.

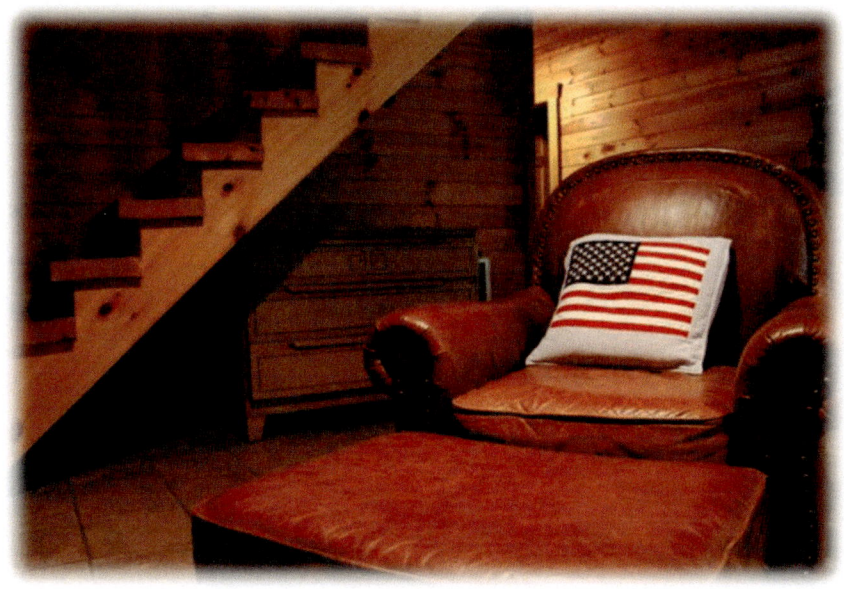

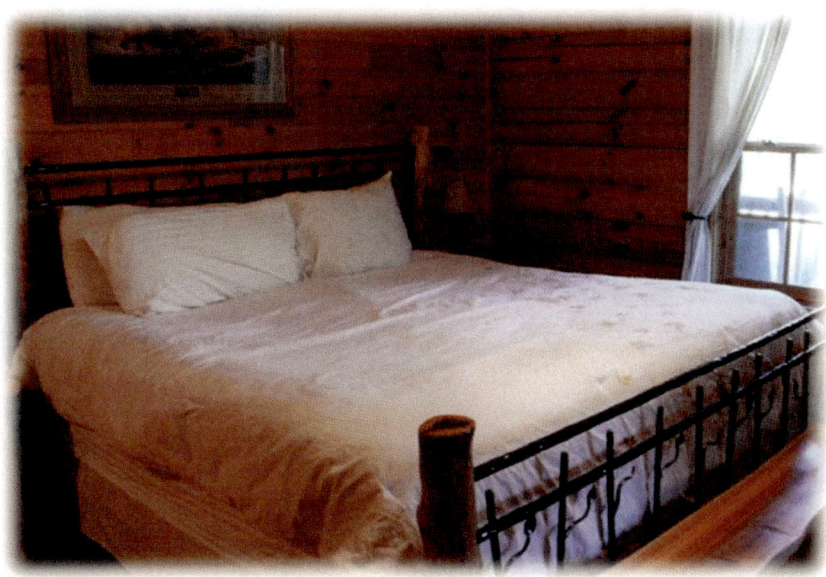

Super Post Workout Shake

This recipe includes cottage cheese - the king of cheap, easy, high BV protein sources! I'll be surprised if you can taste it as the blender smoothes out the texture.

Ingredients

16 oz skim milk

2 cups non-fat cottage cheese

3 scoops vanilla protein

1/2 cup non-fat reduced sugar vanilla yogurt and 1/4 cup of your favorite fruit

8 to 12 drops vanilla

1 handful of ice

Directions

Blend together and chill. Makes (3) 2 cup servings. This is a great post-workout shake. The high-glycemic-value carbs spike insulin to deliver protein to your muscles pronto. Add ¼ cup of dry oats for more complex carbs.

Peanut Butter Chocolate Banana Oatmeal Post Workout Shake

This is my favorite post workout shake. This is not a meal replacement shake. It's a post-training shake and should not be used as a meal replacement shake.

Ingredients

16 oz skim milk

1 banana

3 scoops Chocolate protein

1 table spoon peanut butter

1 table spoon of Agave

¼ cup of Oatmeal

1 Handful of ice

Directions

Blend together and chill. Makes (3) 2 cup servings. This is a great post-workout shake. The high-glycemic-value carbs spike insulin to deliver protein to your muscles pronto. The dry oats add more complex carbs.

A Bit of Green

A super healthy shake that tastes pretty damn good. The flax seed oil helps the nutrients digest gradually so you get a nice slow steady supply of protein. I use agave because it's healthier than sugar. After a workout it will help satisfy your body's need for a simple sugar.

Ingredients

1 cup of pure water
1 scoop of vanilla protein powder
3/4 cup of natural yogurt
1 banana
1 tsp of flax seed oil
2 tsp of Agave
1 tsp Blue green algae

This shake provides carbs, protein and plenty of vitamins and minerals. You can easily use it as a meal replacement.

Note: Generally, I add a tablespoon of psyllium flakes to at least one of my shakes daily for additional fiber. For additional nutrition, you can also add algae to every shake.

Psyllium, is good for your heart. In fact, getting a serving of psyllium a day can reduce your 'bad' (LDL) cholesterol by up to 10%, which in turn can reduce your risk of heart disease by 20%.

Our typical Oasis meal replacement shake looks like this:

A goal of 120 to 200 calories per shake

Ingredients

8 oz of water
a handful of ice
25 grams of protein powder (usually one scoop)
¼ cup of berries of any kind

All Raw

Raw Foods

Raw foods are packed with nutrition and so much fun to make. Come to the Oasis soon and we will prepare some fantastically easy raw food dishes! We use organic raw juices during a detox and the weeks following a detox.

We offer weekend Raw Food's Prep classes for those that do not eat meat. We make raw, vegan and vegetarian meals along with protein meal replacement shakes using David Wolfe's Sun Warrior products.

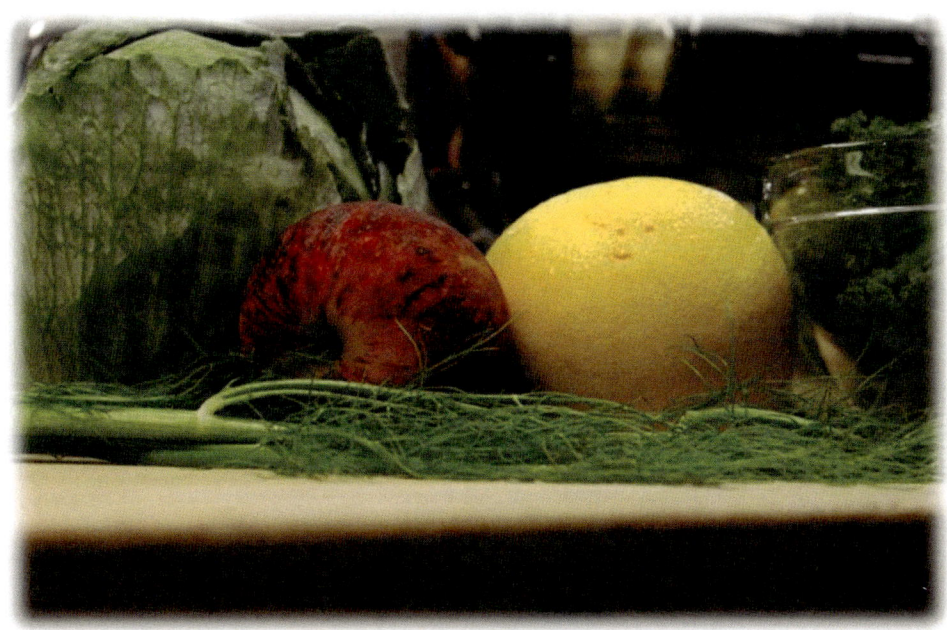

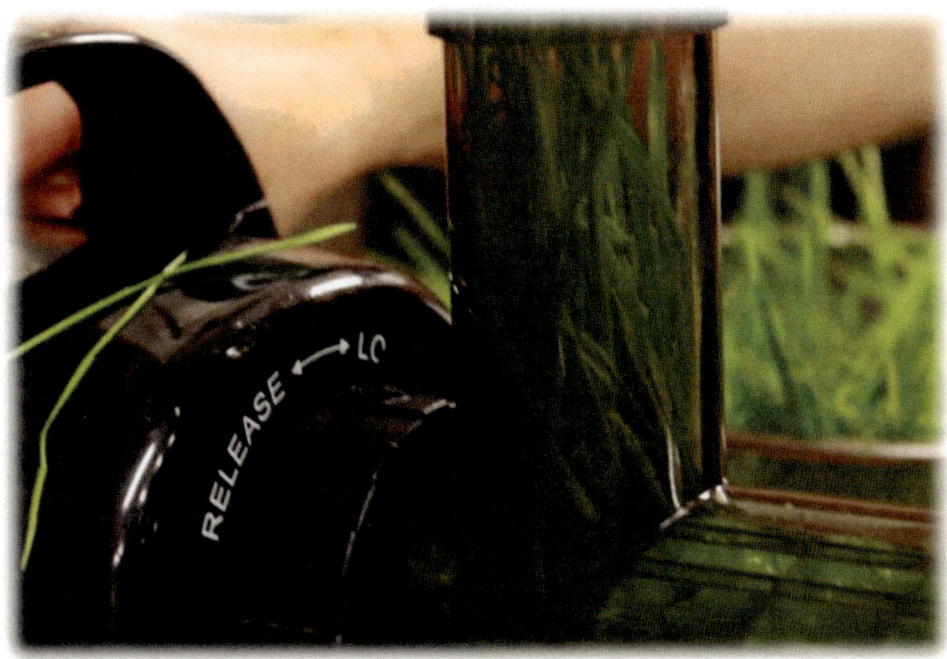

Almond Nut Milk

A fresh healthy drink. As served at DetoxOasis.net.

1	cup	almonds (soaked overnight)	1 tsp	agave (or 4 drops liquid stevia for less calories)
3	cups	water		

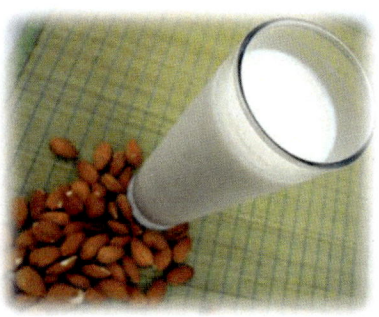

Procedure

6 Soak almonds overnight. Most other nuts take only an hour of soaking.
7 Blend almonds and stevia with water in a Vita-mix or other blender until smooth.
8 Serve.

Equipment Needed:

1 Vita-mix or other strong blender

Servings: 1

Preparation Time: 5 minutes
Cooking Time:
Total Time: 5 minutes

Nutrition Facts

Serving size: Entire recipe (33.7 ounces).

Amount Per Serving	
Calories	842.25
Calories From Fat (72%)	607.81
	% Daily Value
Total Fat 70.67g	109%
Saturated Fat 5.34g	27%
Cholesterol 0mg	0%
Sodium 31.76mg	1%
Potassium 1015.26mg	29%
Total Carbohydrates 30.99g	10%
Fiber 17.45g	70%
Sugar 5.56g	
Protein 30.34g	61%
MyPoints 21.93	

Recipe Tips

Rather than boil your quinoa in just water, try using almond milk, it makes the quinoa really tasty!

Basil Pesto

This is a pesto we serve fresh from our herb garden. As served at FitBodyRetreat.com.

2	cups	fresh basil	1	tsp	nutritional yeast
1/2	cup	macadamia nut oil	1/2	tsp	sea salt*
3	ea	garlic cloves			
1/2	cup	pine nuts (soaked - or any nut you prefer)			

Procedure

1. Put all ingredients in Vita-mix or other blender.
2. Blend and serve.

Equipment Needed:

1. Vita-mix or other strong blender

Servings: 12

Preparation Time: 10 minutes
Cooking Time:
Total Time: 10 minutes

Nutrition Facts

Serving size: 1/12 of a recipe (1.1 ounces).

Amount Per Serving	
Calories	121.37
Calories From Fat (93%)	112.47
	% Daily Value
Total Fat 13.31g	20%
Saturated Fat 0.28g	1%
Cholesterol 0mg	0%
Sodium 79.11mg	3%
Potassium 57.44mg	2%
Total Carbohydrates 1.25g	<1%
Fiber 0.34g	1%
Sugar 0.23g	
Protein 1.12g	2%
MyPoints 3.47	

Recipe Tips

Every summer, I have an herb garden at the ranch. You cannot go wrong with basil, and this recipe is about as raw as you will get. Serve it up with the Mexican Flax Crackers in this cookbook and you will be the pride of the raw food movement!

* Can use Bragg Liquid Aminos as a substitute for salt.

Bean Salad

A spicy bean salad with a kick of lime that is great as a side dish, nacho topping, or all on its own! As served at FitBodyRetreat.com.

14.5	oz	black beans, fresh	1	tsp	cumin
14.5	oz	red kidney beans, fresh	2	tbsp	chili powder
			1	tsp	lime juice
15	oz	garbanzo beans, fresh	4	ea	tomatoes, cubed
14.5	oz	pinto beans, fresh	1	pinch	dried parsley
10	oz	frozen corn, thawed			
1	tbsp	olive oil			

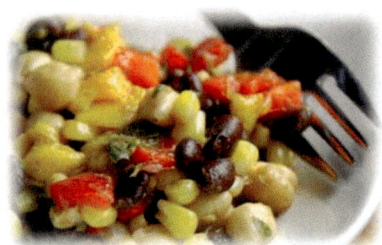

Procedure

1. Cook the beans.
2. Pour beans into a colander and rinse with water.
3. In a large mixing bowl, toss beans and corn together with oil, cumin, chili powder, lime juice and tomato.
4. Sprinkle with parsley, cover and chill.

Servings: 8

Preparation Time: 15 minutes
Cooking Time: 2 minutes
Total Time: 1 hour and 15 minutes

Nutrition Facts

Serving size: 1/8 of a recipe (22.8 ounces).

Amount Per Serving	
Calories	640.98
Calories From Fat (9%)	56.81
	% Daily Value
Total Fat 6.81g	10%
Saturated Fat 0.73g	4%
Cholesterol 0mg	0%
Sodium 51.97mg	2%
Potassium 960.73mg	27%
Total Carbohydrates 130.38g	43%
Fiber 8.99g	36%
Sugar 10.81g	
Protein 27.17g	54%
MyPoints 12.59	

Recipe Tips

Once you hit your fitness and weight loss goals, life is grand! Three meals a day and two protein shakes or bars! Plus, maybe even an extra cheat night is allowed!

Carrot, Apple & Green

This is tasty! It's a drink we don't normally serve here at the ranch because calories and sugar content are high. If we have a guest coming off of alcohol or sugar, they tend to want this type of drink. As served at DetoxOasis.net.

2	ea	carrots	1	ea	cucumber
2	ea	celery stalks	1	ea	apple
1	handful	spinach (about 2 cups)			

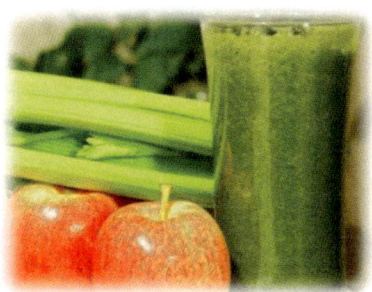

Procedure
1 Blend all ingredients in a Vita-mix or other blender and serve.

Equipment Needed:
1 Vita-mix or other strong blender

Servings: 2

Preparation Time: 5 minutes
Cooking Time:
Total Time: 5 minutes

Nutrition Facts

Serving size: 1/2 of a recipe (14.2 ounces).

Amount Per Serving	
Calories	113.2
Calories From Fat (6%)	6.5
	% Daily Value
Total Fat 0.79g	1%
Saturated Fat 0.11g	<1%
Cholesterol 0mg	0%
Sodium 119.52mg	5%
Potassium 851.6mg	24%
Total Carbohydrates 26.09g	9%
Fiber 6.91g	28%
Sugar 16.38g	
Protein 3.07g	6%
MyPoints 1.53	

Recipe Tips

Anytime you add fruit to something, such as an apple, you add sugar and calories. Most detox centers in the USA won't serve up such a juice. But when I detox, I need more than just green juices on some days. This is a healthy drink any day of the week!

Cocoa Almond Drink

A nice cocoa drink all will enjoy. As served at DetoxOasis.net.

3/4	cup	almond milk	10	drops	liquid vanilla stevia
1	tsp	cocoa powder	2	tsp	extra virgin coconut oil (liquefied*)
1	tsp	agave			

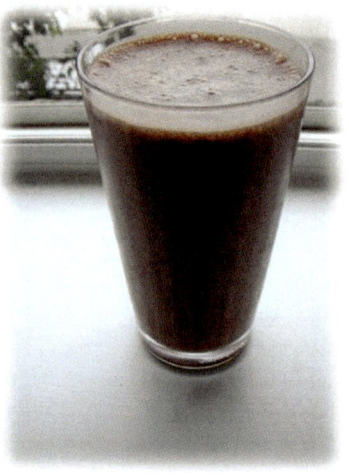

Procedure

1. Blend almond milk, cocoa, agave and stevia in Vita-mix or other blender.
2. Add the coconut oil and blend until smooth and creamy.

Equipment Needed:

1. Vita-mix or other strong blender

Servings: 1

Preparation Time: 5 minutes
Cooking Time:
Total Time: 5 minutes

Nutrition Facts

Serving size: Entire recipe (81.5 ounces).

Amount Per Serving	
Calories	159.84
Calories From Fat (84%)	134.18
	% Daily Value
Total Fat 9.74g	15%
Saturated Fat 0.44g	2%
Cholesterol 0mg	0%
Sodium 118.34mg	5%
Potassium 82.3mg	2%
Total Carbohydrates 3.13g	1%
Fiber 1.79g	7%
Sugar 0.09g	
Protein 1.06g	2%
MyPoints 3.65	

Recipe Tips

One of those raw foodie "rite of passage" drinks.

* Coconut oil must be in liquid form to blend properly.

Dave's Favorite Raw Dressing

A creamy delightful dressing that I learned from a raw enthusiast that passed through our doors here. As served at DetoxOasis.net.

3/4	cup	Tahini	1	ea	lemon, juiced
1/4	cup	Bragg Liquid Aminos	1/4	tsp	sea salt
1/2	cup	apple cider vinegar	1/4	cup	parsley
2	ea	scallions	1/2	cup	water
1	ea	garlic clove			

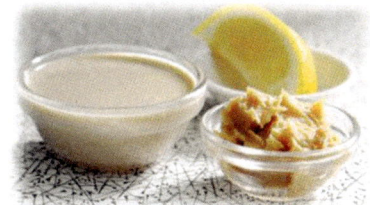

Procedure

1. Add all ingredients to a Vita-mix or other blender and blend well.
2. Serve immediately or refrigerate and serve at a later time.

Equipment Needed:

1. Vita-mix or other strong blender

Servings: 6

Preparation Time: 10 minutes
Cooking Time:
Total Time: 10 minutes

Nutrition Facts

Serving size: 1/6 of a recipe (3.4 ounces).

Amount Per Serving	
Calories	180.72
Calories From Fat (66%)	118.67
	% Daily Value
Total Fat 14.46g	22%
Saturated Fat 2.03g	10%
Cholesterol 0mg	0%
Sodium 424.67mg	18%
Potassium 179.36mg	5%
Total Carbohydrates 9.43g	3%
Fiber 3.05g	12%
Sugar 0.48g	
Protein 7.58g	15%
MyPoints 4.21	

Recipe Tips

One of the nice things about running a center for food and fitness is that you learn a lot of great stuff from others. A raw food chef intern taught me this recipe. It's great!

Energy Soup

A fantastic cold raw soup to break your detox fast with. We make this soup at the ranch. As served at DetoxOasis.net.

2	cups	water	1	ea	apple, large
2	handfuls	spinach (about 4 cups)	2	tbsp	Bragg Liquid Aminos
1/2	cup	sprouts, small handful (any kind)	3	tbsp	carrots, shaved
1/2	cup	almonds, small handful (soaked overnight)	1/8	cup	blueberries
1	ea	dulse seaweed, small piece	2	ea	pear
1	ea	avocado	1	dash	cayenne pepper

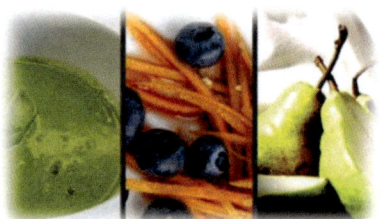

Procedure
1 Set aside a small amount of the carrot, berries and sprouts for a garnish.
2 Add all ingredients except for the pear to a blender. Blend well.
3 Using a large hand grater, grate the pear into a pile.
4 Place the piles of pear into each bowl to create a mountain like appearance.
5 Place the blended cold soup around the mountain of pear.
6 Garnish with a couple of berries and carrots that are cut like a shoe string.
7 Add a few single sprouts.
8 Sprinkle gently with cayenne pepper and serve.

Equipment Needed:
1 Vita-mix or other strong blender

Servings: 6

Preparation Time: 10 minutes
Cooking Time:
Total Time: 10 minutes

Nutrition Facts
Serving size: 1/6 of a recipe (9.6 ounces).

Amount Per Serving	
Calories	180.51
Calories From Fat (47%)	85.38
	% Daily Value
Total Fat 10.57g	16%
Saturated Fat 1.09g	5%
Cholesterol 0mg	0%
Sodium 193.37mg	8%
Potassium 468.74mg	13%
Total Carbohydrates 21.2g	7%
Fiber 6.78g	27%
Sugar 10.81g	
Protein 5.3g	11%
MyPoints 3.69	

Recipe Tips
This is a highly modified version of the Ann Wigmore recipe! If every meal must be an event or must be a taste sensation, then you are condemned to a life of misery, sadness and obesity followed by diabetes and a much shorter life than nature intended for you. Treat food for what it is-- fuel! This dish is really fun fuel! This is the dish we serve our guests on the last day of their detox. It is the first food we serve them as they break their fast.

Ginger Cucumber Salad

A zesty simple plate of cucumbers. As served at FitBodyRetreat.com.

1/3	ea	cucumber, sliced thin	1/2	tsp	oyster sauce
1	tsp	rice wine vinegar	1/4	tsp	hot sauce (Sriracha or rooster sauce)
1	tsp	extra virgin olive oil			
2	tsp	Bragg Liquid Aminos	1/2	tsp	ground ginger
			1	pinch	sea salt

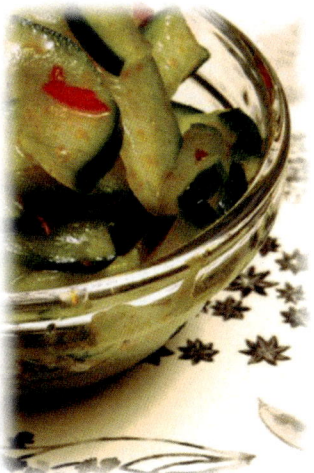

Procedure

1. Slice cucumber thin.
2. Combine remaining ingredients in a bowl except sea salt and mix well.
3. Add cucumbers.
4. Marinate for a few minutes in the refrigerator.
5. Arrange cucumbers nicely on a plate.
6. Add sea salt.

Servings: 1

Preparation Time: 15 minutes
Cooking Time:
Total Time: 30 minutes

Nutrition Facts

Serving size: Entire recipe (4.5 ounces).

Amount Per Serving	
Calories	57.55
Calories From Fat (57%)	32.7
	% Daily Value
Total Fat 4.72g	7%
Saturated Fat 0.66g	3%
Cholesterol 0mg	0%
Sodium 717.8mg	30%
Potassium 191.48mg	5%
Total Carbohydrates 5.33g	2%
Fiber 0.86g	3%
Sugar 1.47g	
Protein 2.74g	5%
MyPoints 1.37	

Recipe Tips

A young lady from Tennessee showed me this dish. It's light, spicy and delicious! Great as a small side or small appetizer.

Green Algae Drink

We serve this drink 4x/day at the ranch. As served at DetoxOasis.net.

1-1/2	tsp	Spirulina blue green algae powder	6	drops	liquid vanilla stevia
1-1/2	cup	water	1	cup	ice
1	ea	lime, juiced			

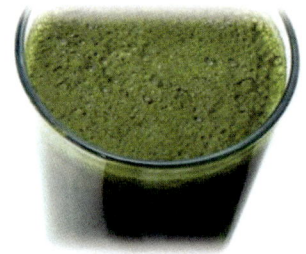

Procedure
1 Mix all together, blend and serve.

Equipment Needed:
1 Vita-mix or other strong blender

Servings: 2

Preparation Time: 4 minutes
Cooking Time:
Total Time: 4 minutes

Nutrition Facts

Serving size: 1/2 of a recipe (20.7 ounces).

Amount Per Serving	
Calories	15.53
Calories From Fat (3%)	0.46
	% Daily Value
Total Fat 0.07g	<1%
Saturated Fat 0.01g	<1%
Cholesterol 0mg	0%
Sodium 8.03mg	<1%
Potassium 35.95mg	1%
Total Carbohydrates 3.91g	1%
Fiber 0.94g	4%
Sugar 0.57g	
Protein 1.21g	2%
MyPoints 0.13	

Recipe Tips

This drink is what I have when I'm fasting or just out of energy. In about 20 minutes, it will regulate your blood sugar, regardless if it's up or down. The reason that I use this drink is it does not cause you nausea like wheat grass can. Wheatgrass is wonderful, but it's very powerful. We train so hard here at our retreat that about 50% of my clients cannot handle the nausea that wheatgrass can produce. So for these clients, it's algae! This recipe was created by my son Rob, and a client of ours, Hap, at one of our Costa Rica retreats.

Green Smoothie & Berries

Refreshing and healthy smoothie. Loaded with minerals, vitamins and taste. As served at DetoxOasis.net.

1	cup	spinach
2	ea	bananas, small
1/2	cup	strawberries (or any berries)
1	ea	orange

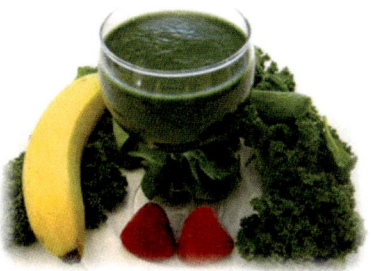

Procedure

1 Put all ingredients in a Vita-mix or other blender and blend until creamy smooth.

Equipment Needed:

1 Vita-mix or other strong blender

Servings: 2

Preparation Time: 5 minutes
Cooking Time: 5 minutes
Total Time: 5 minutes

Nutrition Facts

Serving size: 1/2 of a recipe (8.2 ounces).

Amount Per Serving	
Calories	155.59
Calories From Fat (4%)	5.98
	% Daily Value
Total Fat 0.74g	1%
Saturated Fat 0.16g	<1%
Cholesterol 0mg	0%
Sodium 14.83mg	<1%
Potassium 659.24mg	19%
Total Carbohydrates 38.85g	13%
Fiber 7.29g	29%
Sugar 14.27g	
Protein 2.82g	6%
MyPoints 2.37	

Recipe Tips

If you'd like your smoothie to be even smoother, add an avocado. If sweeter, add mango, pear, coconut, etc.; even a teaspoon of agave. Simple guidelines for any successful smoothie include: anything green - spinach, kale, etc.; any fruit - berries, bananas, peaches, etc.; anything you want - herbs, celery, garlic, sea veggies, etc.

Yes, it's really healthy and pretty tasty. Add a scoop of vanilla protein and it goes from 2 grams to 25 grams of protein! I often add a scoop of protein to my veggie juices simply to reduce the number of items or drinks I consume in a day. Plus, it's faster to only have to clean the blender once.

Green Veggie Juice #1

We serve this drink 2x/day at the ranch. As served at DetoxOasis.net.

1	ea	cucumber	2	ea	celery stalks
2	handfuls	spinach (about 4 cups)	1	dash	cayenne pepper (optional)
1	handful	sprouts (any kind - about 1 cup)			

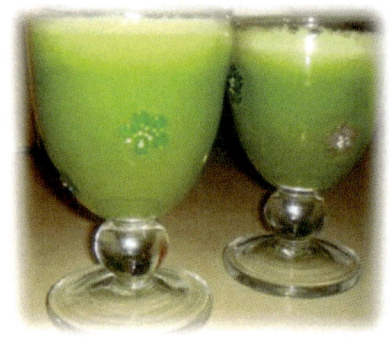

Procedure

1. Mix all ingredients in a Vita-mix blender.
2. Season with cayenne pepper if you'd like to spice it up.
3. Serve and enjoy!

Equipment Needed:

1. Vita-mix or other strong blender

Servings: 1

Preparation Time: 5 minutes
Cooking Time:
Total Time: 5 minutes

Nutrition Facts

Serving size: Entire recipe (21.9 ounces).

Amount Per Serving	
Calories	87.81
Calories From Fat (11%)	9.34
	% Daily Value
Total Fat 1.15g	2%
Saturated Fat 0.16g	<1%
Cholesterol 0mg	0%
Sodium 175.06mg	7%
Potassium 1329.28mg	38%
Total Carbohydrates 14.83g	5%
Fiber 6.3g	25%
Sugar 6.45g	
Protein 6.91g	14%
MyPoints 1.05	

Recipe Tips

Here is a drink I enjoyed at Hippocrates Institute in south Florida. We serve this twice daily during a detox at our fasting and cleansing center, Detox Oasis.

Green Veggie Juice #2

A refreshing juice without a juicer. As served at DetoxOasis.net.

1-1/2	cup	Kale (or spinach)	6	cups	water
2	ea	apples, medium			

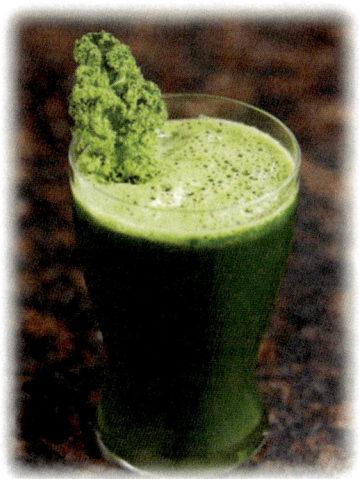

Procedure

1. Blend all ingredients in a Vita-mix or other blender.
2. Pour blended mixture into a nut milk bag.
3. Squeeze mixture over a large bowl and collect the juice.
4. Drink and enjoy!

Equipment Needed:

1. Vita-mix or other strong blender
2. Nut milk bag

Servings: 6

Preparation Time: 5 minutes
Total Time: 5 minutes

Nutrition Facts

Serving size: 1/6 of a recipe (11.1 ounces).

Amount Per Serving		
Calories		39.92
Calories From Fat (4%)		1.76
		% Daily Value
Total Fat 0.22g		<1%
Saturated Fat 0.03g		<1%
Cholesterol 0mg		0%
Sodium 14.92mg		<1%
Potassium 142.16mg		4%
Total Carbohydrates 10.05g		3%
Fiber 1.79g		7%
Sugar 6.3g		
Protein 0.71g		1%
MyPoints 0.46		

Recipe Tips

OK, here is another "Kale Mary, save your life" drink. This drink is so healthy! My only issue with Kale is it does not go through my juicer very well.

Lettuce Veggie Wraps

Raw veggies inside of lettuce wrapped up like a taco. As served at DetoxOasis.net.

2	ea	avocados, ripe	1/4	cup	fresh cilantro, chopped
3	ea	tomatoes, diced	1	ea	kernels from a fresh ear of corn
1/2	ea	jalapeno pepper, diced			
2	tbsp	yellow onion, diced	2	tsp	fresh lime juice
3	ea	garlic cloves, minced	6-8	ea	lettuce leaves

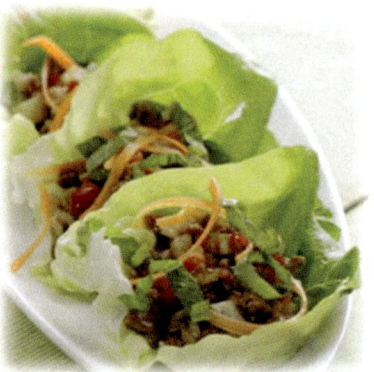

Procedure

1. In a medium sized bowl, mash the avocado.
2. Add remaining ingredients and stir until well mixed.
3. Spread 2-3 tbsp of this mixture onto lettuce leaves and wrap.

Servings: 2

Preparation Time: 20 minutes
Cooking Time:
Total Time: 20 minutes

Nutrition Facts

Serving size: 1/2 of a recipe (18.7 ounces).

Amount Per Serving	
Calories	438.97
Calories From Fat (56%)	247.75
	% Daily Value
Total Fat 30.49g	47%
Saturated Fat 4.42g	22%
Cholesterol 0mg	0%
Sodium 41.61mg	2%
Potassium 1783.52mg	51%
Total Carbohydrates 44.05g	15%
Fiber 18.65g	75%
Sugar 9.99g	
Protein 8.9g	18%
MyPoints 10.52	

Mexican Flax Crackers

Nice crackers that are all raw, not processed! As served at DetoxOasis.net.

3	cups	flax seeds (soaked 2 hrs)	2	tbsp	chili powder
4	med	tomatoes	2	tsp	cilantro, dried
1	ea	red pepper	1	tsp	garlic powder
1/2	cup	Bragg Liquid Aminos			

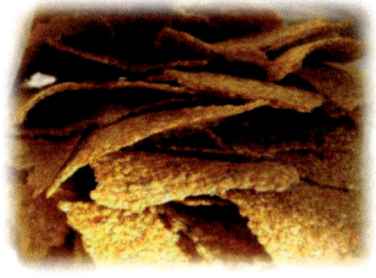

Procedure

1. Soak the flax seeds in 6 cups of water for 4-6 hours.
2. Blend the tomatoes and red pepper in a Vita-mix or other blender.
3. Add the rest of the ingredients to the Vita-mix.
4. Spread the mixture as thin as possible on a teflex sheet - about 1/4" thick.
5. Set in dehydrator at 105 degrees for 5-6 hours.
6. Flip the cracker over and remove teflex sheet.
7. Continue to dehydrate for another 4-5 hours or until completely dry.

Equipment Needed:

1. Vita-mix or other strong blender
2. Dehydrator

Servings: 4

Preparation Time: 30 minutes
Cooking Time: 12 hours
Total Time: 12 hours

Nutrition Facts

Serving size: 1/4 of a recipe (12.8 ounces).

Amount Per Serving	
Calories	619.61
Calories From Fat (62%)	384.66
	% Daily Value
Total Fat 42.21g	65%
Saturated Fat 0.15g	<1%
Cholesterol 0mg	0%
Sodium 1076.33mg	45%
Potassium 488.13mg	14%
Total Carbohydrates 47.53g	16%
Fiber 3.87g	15%
Sugar 5.38g	
Protein 10.48g	21%
MyPoints 15.14	

Recipe Tips

If you keep your hands wet, the mixture seems to spread easier. Generally, when I prepare smoky raw cheese, I also make these crackers to go with the yummy cheese. Make sure you dehydrate these well. If they are soft, they just don't digest well.

Pico-de-Gallo

Here is a nice fresh topping for beans, egg dishes, burritos or quinoa. As served at FitBodyRetreat.com.

1/2	cup	tomatoes, seeded and diced	2	ea	limes, juiced
1/4	cup	red onion, diced	2	tbsp	cilantro (plus extra for garnish)
1	tbsp	jalapenos, diced, seeds removed	2	tbsp	Bragg Liquid Aminos
1	tbsp	garlic, minced	1	pinch	black pepper

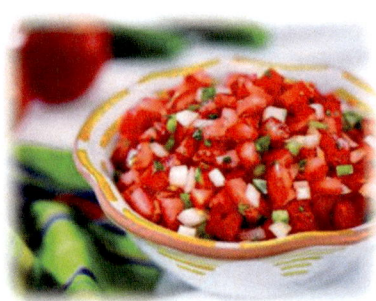

Procedure

1. Mix all in a bowl and place atop your favorite dish or serve with our High Protein Chips or Mexican Flax Crackers.

Servings: 2

Preparation Time: 15 minutes
Cooking Time:
Total Time: 15 minutes

Nutrition Facts

Serving size: 1/2 of a recipe (4.8 ounces).

Amount Per Serving	
Calories	50.48
Calories From Fat (13%)	6.45
	% Daily Value
Total Fat 1.09g	2%
Saturated Fat 0.08g	<1%
Cholesterol 0mg	0%
Sodium 486.51mg	20%
Potassium 254.82mg	7%
Total Carbohydrates 11.93g	4%
Fiber 3.42g	14%
Sugar 2.1g	
Protein 4.81g	10%
MyPoints 0.42	

Recipe Tips

This is great on so many dishes. Great with the Mexican Flax Crackers! Great on omelets! Great with a salad!

* See recipe for High Protein Chips or Mexican Flax Crackers

Raw-Alfredo Sauce

A perfect topping for spaghetti squash or peeled zucchini! As served at DetoxOasis.net.

2	cups	cashews (soaked 2 hrs)	1	tsp	onion powder
1/4	cup	Bragg Liquid Aminos	2/3	cup	water
2	tsp	nutritional yeast	1	pinch	sea salt
1	ea	garlic clove			

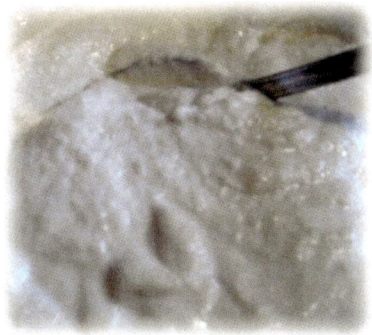

Procedure

1 In a Vita-mix or other blender, add all ingredients and blend until smooth.
2 Serve as desired.

Equipment Needed:

1 Vita-mix or other strong blender

Servings: 4

Preparation Time: 10 minutes
Cooking Time:
Total Time: 10 minutes

Nutrition Facts

Serving size: 1/4 of a recipe (4.2 ounces).

Amount Per Serving	
Calories	86.05
Calories From Fat (56%)	48.56
	% Daily Value
Total Fat 6.73g	10%
Saturated Fat 1.11g	6%
Cholesterol 0mg	0%
Sodium 555.64mg	23%
Potassium 102.87mg	3%
Total Carbohydrates 5.5g	2%
Fiber 0.57g	2%
Sugar 0.89g	
Protein 6.19g	12%
MyPoints 2.17	

Recipe Tips

This is way better than what you will find processed in a jar! Put this on your zucchini slices or your rice pasta. You will love it!

Raw-Apple Sauce

A good sweet dessert that's fresh and 100% raw. As served at DetoxOasis.net.

- 2 ea apples, large (any sweet variety)
- 2 ea dates (any sweet variety like Medjool)
- 1/2 tsp cinnamon

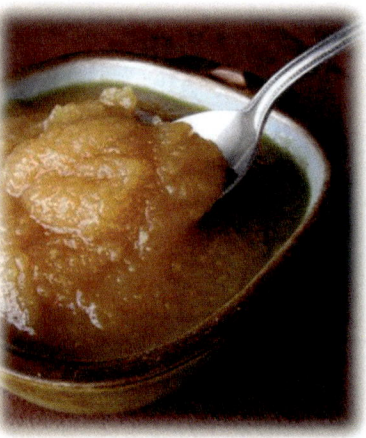

Procedure

1. Cut up the apples into smaller chunks.
2. Place apples, dates and cinnamon in a food processor using the "S" blade.
3. Pulse until chunky but well mixed.

Equipment Needed:

1. Food processor

Servings: 2

Preparation Time: 10 minutes
Cooking Time:
Total Time: 10 minutes

Nutrition Facts

Serving size: 1/2 of a recipe (11.4 ounces).

Amount Per Serving	
Calories	178.57
Calories From Fat (2%)	3.08
	% Daily Value
Total Fat 0.39g	<1%
Saturated Fat 0.06g	<1%
Cholesterol 0mg	0%
Sodium 2.3mg	<1%
Potassium 241.41mg	7%
Total Carbohydrates 49.32g	16%
Fiber 5.7g	23%
Sugar 23.18g	
Protein 0.61g	1%
MyPoints 2.8	

Recipe Tips

Somehow, when I eat this, it just feels "right". How much easier and more natural can it get! Don't forget --calories are calories, raw or not. Make sure you know your numbers and never try to justify high calorie foods by saying "at least it's healthy".

Raw-Berry Cheesecake

100% raw dessert. A delicious cheesecake alternative! As served at DetoxOasis.net.

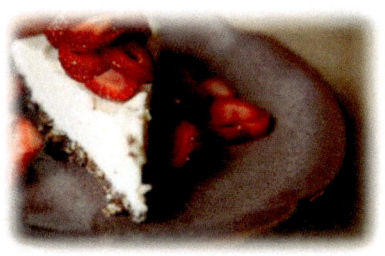

Crust
- 1-1/2 cup almonds (soaked overnight)
- 1 cup raisins

Filling
- 3 cup cashews (soaked 2 hrs)
- 1 cup lemon juice
- 1 cup honey
- 1 cup extra virgin coconut oil
- 1 tsp almond extract

Topping
- 1 bag frozen strawberries (or any other berries, 16-20 oz bag)
- 1/4 cup agave

Procedure

Crust
1. Mix the raisins and almonds in the food processor until fine.
2. Press this mixture into a pie plate.
3. Place in refrigerator.

Filling
1. Blend cashews, lemon juice, honey, coconut oil and almond extract in a Vita-mix or other strong blender.
2. Pour this mixture onto the crust.
3. Put the pie back into the refrigerator for 2+ hrs.
4. Serve after chilled.

Topping
1. Blend the frozen berries and agave in the Vita-mix blender.
2. Pour the topping onto each piece of pie as it is served.
3. Keep topping separate from whole pie and in refrigerator until served.

Equipment Needed:
1. Vita-mix or other strong blender
2. Food processor

Servings: 8

Preparation Time: 30 minutes
Cooking Time:
Total Time: 2 hours and 30 minutes

Nutrition Facts

Serving size: 1/8 of a recipe (8.3 ounces).

Amount Per Serving		
Calories		883.48
Calories From Fat (58%)		509.44
		% Daily Value
Total Fat 58.94g		91%
Saturated Fat 0.03g		<1%
Cholesterol 0mg		0%
Sodium 10.88mg		<1%
Potassium 312.83mg		9%
Total Carbohydrates 83.07g		28%
Fiber 2.43g		10%
Sugar 51.01g		
Protein 14.3g		29%
MyPoints 22.1		

Recipe Tips

You won't find many dessert recipes in my cookbook. Why? Because with me, it's either dessert or wine after dinner. You must choose one! It can never be both. "Please pass the Shiraz!" Note: This cheesecake is crazy good!

Raw-Chocolate Avocado Mousse

Creamy, rich, and completely raw. Your guests will be shocked when they learn it's a raw dessert!

- 4 ea   avocados, ripe
- 1 cup   agave (or evaporated cane juice)
- 1 tbsp   vanilla extract
- 1 cup   cocoa powder, organic fair trade (or carob)

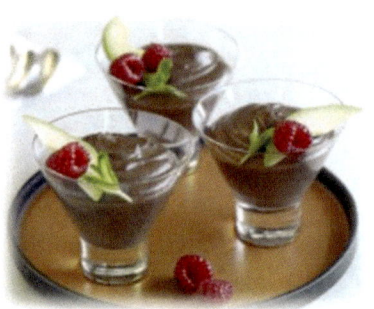

Procedure

1. Slice each avocado open and scoop out the insides.
2. Place the avocado meat in a food processor or blender.
3. Add the agave, vanilla and cocoa powder.
4. Blend or process the mixture until fully blended.
5. Mixture should be smooth and the color of chocolate.
6. Can be served instantly, but tastes better after being refrigerated for at least 1 hr.
7. Serve in small cups with fresh fruit* or a sprig of mint on top - like a peppermint piece you find in some ice cream.

Equipment Needed:

1. Vita-mix or other strong blender, or a food processor

Servings: 4

Preparation Time: 10 minutes
Cooking Time:
Total Time: 1 hour and 15 minutes

Nutrition Facts

Serving size: 1/4 of a recipe (8.8 ounces).

Amount Per Serving	
Calories	559.98
Calories From Fat (45%)	253.44
	% Daily Value
Total Fat 32.41g	50%
Saturated Fat 6.01g	30%
Cholesterol 0mg	0%
Sodium 18.88mg	<1%
Potassium 1307.32mg	37%
Total Carbohydrates 78g	26%
Fiber 20.61g	82%
Sugar 2.11g	
Protein 8.24g	16%
MyPoints 13.1	

Recipe Tips

I was taught this dessert by a good friend, Kat from Bloomington, Indiana. She is working on a project called Spirit Tree Farms. She is into all sorts of funky stuff. This tastes great! But I have to say "no thank you my dear, I'm saving my calories for the wine!" It's the reality and a shame. Unfortunately, it's got to be one or the other after the age of 40.

* Good fruits to top this with are strawberries, raspberries, blueberries, and sometimes pineapple.

Raw-Fajita Alternative

A great alternative to the standard fajita. As service at DetoxOasis.net.

2	ea	portabella mushroom caps	1/3	cup	Bragg Liquid Aminos
1	ea	red onion, medium	1/4	cup	cumin
1	ea	red pepper	4	ea	lettuce leaves, large (or Collard, Romaine, etc.)
1	ea	yellow bell pepper			
3/4	cup	extra virgin olive oil			

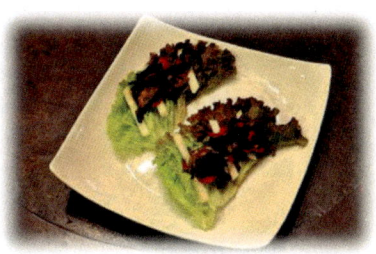

Procedure

1. Slice peppers, mushrooms and onion into long thin strips.
2. Mix all ingredients in a bowl except for lettuce leaves.
3. Pour mixture into a zip lock bag.
4. Refrigerate this marinated mix for 6 hrs, turning bag often.
5. Serve the marinated mix in the lettuce leaves. Wrap up like a fajita.

Servings: 4

Preparation Time: 20 minutes
Cooking Time: 6 hours
Total Time: 6 hours and 30 minutes

Nutrition Facts

Serving size: 1/4 of a recipe (9.2 ounces).

Amount Per Serving	
Calories	431.2
Calories From Fat (82%)	353.85
	% Daily Value
Total Fat 42.37g	65%
Saturated Fat 5.76g	29%
Cholesterol 0mg	0%
Sodium 664.17mg	28%
Potassium 573.15mg	16%
Total Carbohydrates 12.9g	4%
Fiber 3.38g	14%
Sugar 3.75g	
Protein 7.94g	16%
MyPoints 11.48	

Recipe Tips

There are really good. What makes or breaks this dish is the onion. Try and go with a sweet Vidalia onion. If the onion is too hot, it overpowers the dish and then it's just too much onion flavor.

Raw-Garden Burgers

This recipe brings the garden to the burger! As served at DetoxOasis.net.

6 tbsp	water	
3 tbsp	flax seeds, ground	
1 handful	parsley, fresh (or 4 tbsp fresh or 4 tsp dried)	
1 cup	carrot pulp*	
1 cup	shelled sunflower seeds, ground	
1/2 cup	celery, finely chopped	
6 tbsp	green onion, chopped	
2 tbsp	red pepper, chopped	
2 tsp	Bragg Liquid Aminos	

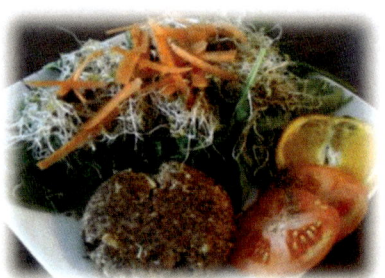

Procedure

1. Grind flax seeds in a coffee grinder.
2. In your Vita-mix or blender - combine the water and the ground flax seeds and blend well.
3. Pour mixture into a bowl - set aside.
4. In a separate bowl - mix carrot pulp, sunflower seeds, parsley, celery, onion, pepper and liquid aminos.
5. Add flax seed mixture to other ingredients.
6. Form into 6 patties about 1/2" thick. (if you need more water, add enough to make a good patty)
7. Dehydrate at 110 degrees for 4-8 hours.

Equipment Needed:

1. Coffee grinder
2. Vita-mix or other strong blender
3. Dehydrator

Servings: 6

Preparation Time: 30 minutes
Cooking Time: 8 hours
Total Time: 8 hours

Nutrition Facts

Serving size: 1/6 of a recipe (2.5 ounces).

Amount Per Serving	
Calories	89.8
Calories From Fat (61%)	54.45
	% Daily Value
Total Fat 6.58g	10%
Saturated Fat 0.58g	3%
Cholesterol 0mg	0%
Sodium 79.46mg	3%
Potassium 220.86mg	6%
Total Carbohydrates 6.13g	2%
Fiber 3.28g	13%
Sugar 1.64g	
Protein 3.48g	7%
MyPoints 1.69	

Recipe Tips

Veggie burgers are a great alternative to meat. Just make sure you drink a protein shake with it to maintain your desired protein levels.

* To make carrot pulp - juice some carrots and use the pulp that is remaining.

Raw-Ice Cream Sundae

What can I say? It's ice cream. As served at DetoxOasis.net.

The Base
2 ea frozen bananas

The Sauce
2 tbsp agave
1-1/2 tsp cocoa powder
1 dash almond extract

The Toppings
1 ea dates
1 tbsp walnuts finely chopped (or any nut)
1/4 cup fresh raspberries (optional, or any fruit)

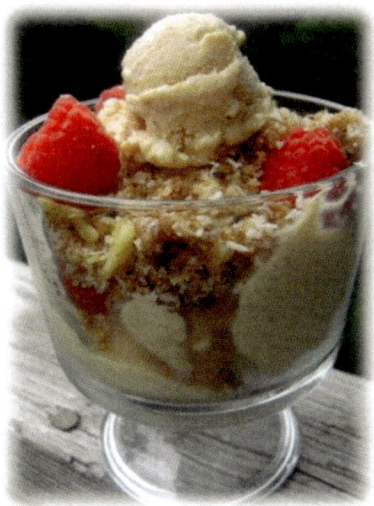

Procedure
1. Blend bananas in Vita-mix or other blender until smooth.
2. Mix agave, cocoa and almond extract in a separate bowl and pour over the banana puree.
3. Add the toppings and serve.

Equipment Needed:
1. Vita-mix or other strong blender

Servings: 2

Preparation Time: 10 minutes
Cooking Time:
Total Time: 10 minutes

Nutrition Facts
Serving size: 1/2 of a recipe (16.8 ounces).

Amount Per Serving	
Calories	218.95
Calories From Fat (66%)	145.54
	% Daily Value
Total Fat 42.12g	65%
Saturated Fat 0.56g	3%
Cholesterol 0mg	0%
Sodium 29.16mg	1%
Potassium 128.69mg	4%
Total Carbohydrates 34.81g	12%
Fiber 2.93g	12%
Sugar 3.48g	
Protein 3.15g	6%
MyPoints 7.3	

Recipe Tips
Raw foods are interesting, and most often, very healthy and nutritious. Even more interesting is the cult-like following the raw food movement seems to have!

Raw-Oatmeal Cookies

2 cups	oat groats, whole	1/2 cup agave (or maple syrup)
1/2 cup	almonds	1/4 cup cashews
1/2 cup	raisins	

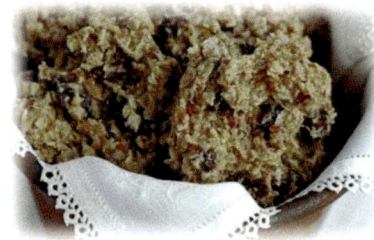

Procedure

1. Put oats in food processor and grind until fine.
2. Transfer to a mixing bowl.
3. Put almonds in food processor and pulse a few times to chop them until just coarsely chopped.
4. Transfer to bowl with the groats.
5. Add raisins and agave to bowl and mix everything well.
6. Grind cashews in a coffee grinder.
7. Use this to coat your palms as you handle the cookie dough.
8. Take small chunks of dough and flatten into round cookie shapes onto the mesh sheet of a dehydrator tray.
9. Dehydrate for about 12 hrs on 110 degrees. Dehydrating time will vary depending on how thick you've made your cookies and the desired chewy/crunchiness.

Equipment Needed:

1. Food processor
2. Coffee Grinder
3. Dehydrator

Servings: 6

Preparation Time: 20 minutes
Cooking Time: 24 hours
Total Time: 24 hours

Nutrition Facts

Serving size: 1/6 of a recipe (3.3 ounces).

Amount Per Serving	
Calories	374.82
Calories From Fat (21%)	77.06
	% Daily Value
Total Fat 9.43g	15%
Saturated Fat 0.78g	4%
Cholesterol 0mg	0%
Sodium 8.15mg	<1%
Potassium 361.93mg	10%
Total Carbohydrates 71.78g	24%
Fiber 7.59g	30%
Sugar 8.6g	
Protein 10.2g	20%
MyPoints 7.48	

Recipe Tips

You can add a couple scoops of chocolate protein powder to this for high protein raw cookies. Be careful though! It's hard to eat just a couple!

Raw-Ranch Dressing

Wonderful alternative to your typical ranch dressing. 100% raw and tastes great! As served at DetoxOasis.net.

1-1/2	cups	cashews or macadamia nuts (soaked 2 hrs)	1	tsp	garlic powder	
			3	tsp	onion powder	
			1-1/2	tsp	dill	
3/4	cup	water	1	tbsp	sea salt	
3	tbsp	lemon juice	1/2	tsp	dried basil	
1/3	cup	apple cider vinegar				
1/3	cup	extra virgin olive oil				
3	tbsp	agave				
2	ea	garlic cloves				

Set Aside

1/4	cup	parsley, finely minced
1/2	tsp	dill

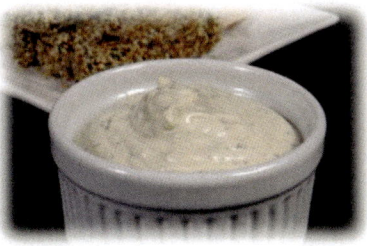

Procedure

1. After soaking nuts, blend all ingredients in a Vita-mix or other blender, except those ingredients set aside.
2. Stir in the set aside ingredients with a large spoon after you are done blending, and serve.

Equipment Needed:

1. Vita-mix or other strong blender

Servings: 8

Preparation Time: 20 minutes
Cooking Time:
Total Time: 20 minutes

Nutrition Facts

Serving size: 1/8 of a recipe (6.5 ounces).

Amount Per Serving	
Calories	232.47
Calories From Fat (74%)	172.75
	% Daily Value
Total Fat 18.05g	28%
Saturated Fat 1.25g	6%
Cholesterol 0mg	0%
Sodium 1181.94mg	49%
Potassium 43.66mg	1%
Total Carbohydrates 7.94g	3%
Fiber 0.33g	1%
Sugar 0.24g	
Protein 6.1g	12%
MyPoints 6.09	

Raw-Smokey Jalapeno Cheese Alternative

Here is a cheese alternative that's easy to make and has great flavor. As served at DetoxOasis.net.

3	cups	cashews (soaked 2 hrs)	2	ea	jalapeno (remove seeds)
3	capsules	granular type probiotics	1	pinch	onion powder
			1	pinch	garlic powder
2/3	cups	rejuvelac*	1	pinch	sea salt
1/2	ea	lemon, juiced	1/2	tsp	nutritional yeast
1/2	ea	tomato, medium	1	tbsp	liquid smoke
1/2	ea	red pepper			

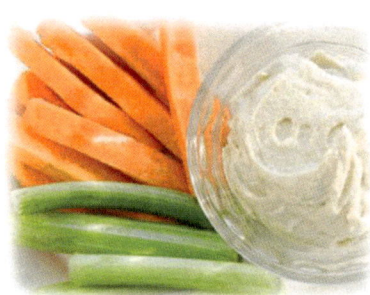

Procedure

1. Mix all ingredients in Vita-mix or other blender until smooth.
2. Line a strainer with a cheesecloth.
3. Set the cheese mixture on to the cheesecloth.
4. Cover the cheese mixture.
5. Store in room temperature for 14-16 hrs.
6. Shape into whatever form you desire.
7. Place in refrigerator for 4 hrs wrapped in plastic.
8. Serve with carrot sticks, celery, or your favorite cracker.

Equipment Needed:

1. Vita-mix or other strong blender

Servings: 20

Preparation Time: 20 minutes
Cooking Time: 20 hours
Total Time: 20 hours

Nutrition Facts

Serving size: 1/20 of a recipe (1.7 ounces).

Amount Per Serving	
Calories	102.37
Calories From Fat (66%)	67.23
	% Daily Value
Total Fat 7.33g	11%
Saturated Fat 0.01g	<1%
Cholesterol 0mg	0%
Sodium 27.01mg	1%
Potassium 18.89mg	<1%
Total Carbohydrates 5.48g	2%
Fiber 0.18g	<1%
Sugar 0.29g	
Protein 3.14g	6%
MyPoints 2.62	

Recipe Tips

Raw foods can be good for you, or they can be just "way too many calories". Listed in this book are a few fun raw dishes to try. You can decide for yourself, based on taste, time to prepare these dishes, and the calorie counts associated with each dish, if they are going to be part of your daily diet. You will love this cheese. I guarantee it! It's fun to make, and your friends won't believe it's raw!

*Rejuvelac is the liquid leftover from soaking wheat grass seeds. You can learn more about making rejuvelac by visiting our Growing Sprouts and Making Rejuvelac recipe.

Raw-Sour Cream

This raw sour cream tastes awesome! As served at DetoxOasis.net.

1	cup	cashews (soaked 2 hrs)	1/4	cup	water
1/4	cup	lemon juice			

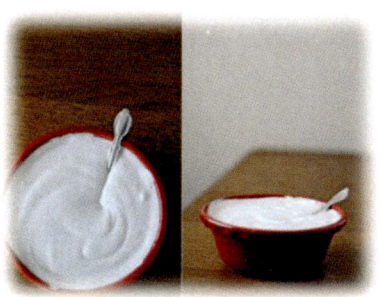

Procedure

1. Add all ingredients to a Vita-mix or other blender.
2. Blend until really creamy.
3. Refrigerate for 2 hrs and then serve.

Equipment Needed:

1. Vita-mix or other strong blender

Servings: 12

Preparation Time: 10 minutes
Cooking Time:
Total Time: 2 hours and 10 minutes

Nutrition Facts

Serving size: 1/12 of a recipe (0.6 ounces).

Amount Per Serving	
Calories	55.45
Calories From Fat (66%)	36.46
	% Daily Value
Total Fat 4.01g	6%
Saturated Fat 0g	0%
Cholesterol 0mg	0%
Sodium 1.2mg	<1%
Potassium 5.29mg	<1%
Total Carbohydrates 3.02g	1%
Fiber 0.02g	<1%
Sugar 0.13g	
Protein 1.68g	3%
MyPoints 1.44	

Recipe Tips

Included in these pages are many raw food recipes. Many of them are fun and healthy. Many of them, in my opinion, are just not worth the calories. I've included the calorie counts for you to make your own decision on what is acceptable to you. Remember to add high fat and high carbs on your cheat day! You must trick that fat storing device of yours!

Raw-Taco's Tasty Meat Alternative

A great raw taco filler. As served at DetoxOasis.net.

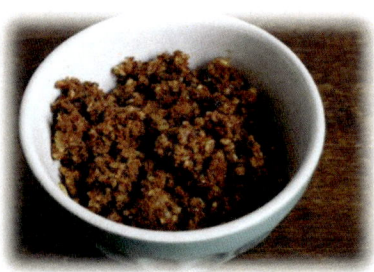

Meat
- 1-1/2 cups walnuts, ground
- 1-1/2 tsp cumin
- 2 tsp taco seasoning
- 2 tsp Bragg Liquid Aminos
- 1/4 tsp cayenne pepper

Toppings
- 2 ea tomatoes
- 2 tbsp fresh cilantro
- 1/2 cup cheese, low fat (or fat free) or raw alternative
- 2 handfuls spinach
- 1/2 cup hot sauce*

Wrap
- 4 ea Ezekiel 4:9 sprouted grain tortillas

Procedure
1. Pulse the walnuts in a food processor gently until ground.
2. Add remaining meat ingredients and continue to pulse on and off. The idea here is to create a chunky meat like filler. If you pulse too long, it will end up being just a creamy mess.
3. Place cheese on the tortillas and melt in oven.
4. Add remaining toppings. Roll up taco and serve.

Equipment Needed:
1. Food processor

Servings: 4

Preparation Time: 10 minutes
Cooking Time:
Total Time: 10 minutes

Nutrition Facts
Serving size: 1/4 of a recipe (12.6 ounces).

Amount Per Serving	
Calories	419.96
Calories From Fat (50%)	210.51
	% Daily Value
Total Fat 25.05g	39%
Saturated Fat 2.59g	13%
Cholesterol 2.97mg	<1%
Sodium 1222.85mg	51%
Potassium 1183.12mg	34%
Total Carbohydrates 36.24g	12%
Fiber 6.17g	25%
Sugar 2.22g	
Protein 19.84g	40%
MyPoints 9.69	

Recipe Tips
Here is my favorite raw recipe. Simple, fast, and yummy! I serve this dish at least once a week. Erica, from Chicago, taught me this dish. I'll suspect one day she will be a well-known author or advocate. She is a talented writer and chef.

* I like Cholula Hot Sauce!

Raw-Zucchini Pasta

A simple pasta alternative with our Spaghetti Sauce or Raw Alfredo Sauce. As served at DetoxOasis.net.

1 ea zucchini, raw

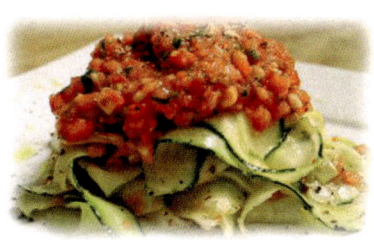

Procedure

1. Peel the skin off the zucchini with a vegetable peeler.
2. Peel the zucchini down to the seeds.
3. Place the peelings in a bowl.
4. Serve with our Spaghetti Sauce or Raw Alfredo Sauce.

Servings: 1

Preparation Time: 5 minutes
Cooking Time: 5 minutes
Total Time: 5 minutes

Nutrition Facts

Serving size: Entire recipe (6.9 ounces).

Amount Per Serving	
Calories	33.32
Calories From Fat (16%)	5.33
	% Daily Value
Total Fat 0.63g	<1%
Saturated Fat 0.16g	<1%
Cholesterol 0mg	0%
Sodium 15.68mg	<1%
Potassium 511.56mg	15%
Total Carbohydrates 6.1g	2%
Fiber 1.96g	8%
Sugar 4.9g	
Protein 2.37g	5%
MyPoints 0.33	

Recipe Tips

I love raw foods! But I also eat a balance of cooked foods. My rule of thumb is this: when I meet someone who looks amazing, I like to ask them about their diet. It is the person that looks amazing that you will learn the most from regarding how you, too, may improve your diet and your look! Take a look at the raw foodie Jenna Norwood down Sarasota way. She's quite possibly one of the fittest and sexiest raw ladies out there. She has some amazing videos and books published. Check out her work. Kelly Serbonich, former chef at Hippocrates Institute in South Florida, first introduced me to raw pasta here at my ranch in Indiana. Together, we did a short local television show on raw foods.

Real Orange & Fresh

Yummy fresh and sweet! Delicious and fresh! As served at DetoxOasis.net.

1	cup	fresh squeezed orange juice	1/2 cup	ice
5	drops	liquid stevia, vanilla		

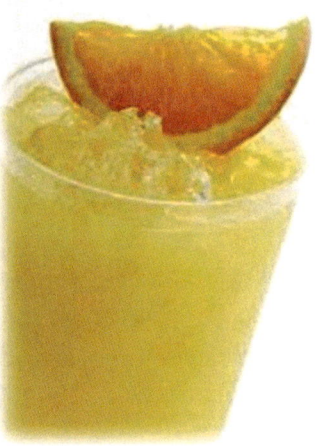

Procedure

1. Peel and juice the oranges.
2. Blend all ingredients using a blender or juicer.

Equipment Needed:

1. Vita-mix or other strong blender, or juicer

Servings: 1

Preparation Time: 5 minutes
Cooking Time:
Total Time: 5 minutes

Nutrition Facts

Serving size: Entire recipe (28.1 ounces).

Amount Per Serving	
Calories	111.6
Calories From Fat (4%)	4.38
	% Daily Value
Total Fat 0.5g	<1%
Saturated Fat 0.06g	<1%
Cholesterol 0mg	0%
Sodium 2.48mg	<1%
Potassium 496mg	14%
Total Carbohydrates 25.79g	9%
Fiber 0.5g	2%
Sugar 20.83g	
Protein 1.74g	3%
MyPoints 2.17	

Seaweed Mineral Drink

A bold RAW drink we serve at the ranch. Loaded with vitamins and minerals. This recipe was brought to us by Kat, a friend and occasionally our raw food chef from Bloomington, Indiana. As served at DetoxOasis.net.

1	ea	apple		1	tbsp	kelp
1	ea	orange		1/2	tsp	garlic
3	ea	dates		1/2	ea	banana
2	tbsp	Spirulina blue green algae powder		1	tbsp	agave
2	tbsp	chlorella				

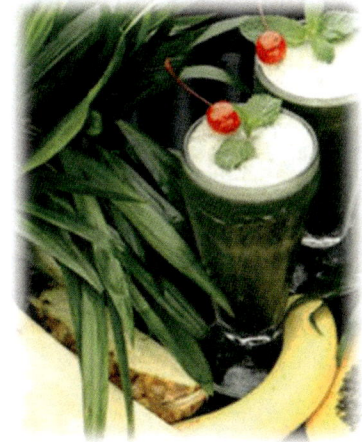

Procedure

1. Place all items in Vita-mix or other blender.
2. Blend well and serve.

Equipment Needed:

1. Vita-mix or other strong blender

Servings: 2

Preparation Time: 5 minutes
Cooking Time:
Total Time: 5 minutes

Nutrition Facts

Serving size: 1/2 of a recipe (20 ounces).

Amount Per Serving	
Calories	239.79
Calories From Fat (2%)	5.44
	% Daily Value
Total Fat 0.56g	<1%
Saturated Fat 0.1g	<1%
Cholesterol 0mg	0%
Sodium 30.59mg	1%
Potassium 445.5mg	13%
Total Carbohydrates 42.94g	14%
Fiber 7.57g	30%
Sugar 20.97g	
Protein 11.38g	23%
MyPoints 4.04	

Recipe Tips

If I was told I only had a few months to live, there are certain foods I would turn to. Just about 100% of them are raw. Raw foods are clean and pure and will heal you, if used correctly. Don't let my occasional negative attitude regarding raw foodists say otherwise. This recipe is one of those, "serious fuel, little fun, high nutrition, save your ass when you are pronounced dying", drinks. Recipe from Kat, friend and client at Spirit Tree Farms in Bloomington, Indiana.

Spicy Fruity Thai Sensation

A delicious, fruity, sweet, sour, hot dish that was created here at the ranch using proven Thai cooking principles. As served at FitBodyRetreat.com.

2	tbsp	oyster sauce	1	ea	pear
1	tbsp	Bragg Liquid Aminos	1	ea	avocado
1	tbsp	hot sauce (Sriracha or rooster sauce)	1	ea	mango
4	tbsp	agave	1	ea	lemon, juiced

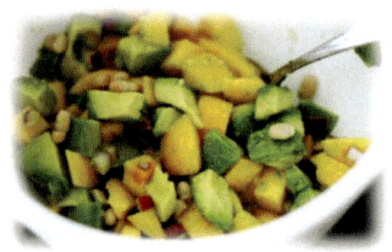

Procedure

1. Cut up fruit into small squares.
2. Combine all ingredients into a bowl or container with lid.
3. Squeeze the juice from 1 lemon onto it.
4. Shake or stir all together. (I prefer to shake)
5. Serve in a small cocktail dish.

Servings: 6

Preparation Time: 10 minutes
Cooking Time:
Total Time: 10 minutes

Nutrition Facts

Serving size: 1/6 of a recipe (11.1 ounces).

Amount Per Serving	
Calories	131.55
Calories From Fat (41%)	53.68
	% Daily Value
Total Fat 4.66g	7%
Saturated Fat 0.65g	3%
Cholesterol 0mg	0%
Sodium 327.14mg	14%
Potassium 256.22mg	7%
Total Carbohydrates 13.62g	5%
Fiber 3.49g	14%
Sugar 7.98g	
Protein 1.59g	3%
MyPoints 2.32	

Recipe Tips

See why wine is good for you? I created this delicious recipe after being over-served on some red wine one night with clients at the Oasis! You will love it. Sweet, sour, hot, and spicy!

Veggies & Hummus Dip

As served at FitBodyRetreat.com.

1/2	cup	broccoli tops	5	ea	cherry tomatoes
6	ea	carrot sticks	1/4	cup	hummus

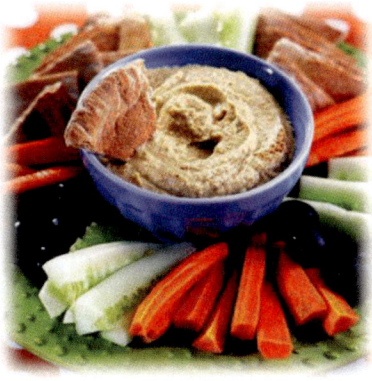

Procedure

1 Arrange vegetables on a plate and serve with hummus as dip.

Servings: 1

Preparation Time: 5 minutes
Cooking Time:
Total Time: 5 minutes

Nutrition Facts

Serving size: Entire recipe (23.8 ounces).

Amount Per Serving	
Calories	335.6
Calories From Fat (17%)	57.72
	% Daily Value
Total Fat 6.82g	10%
Saturated Fat 0.9g	5%
Cholesterol 0mg	0%
Sodium 500.89mg	21%
Potassium 1963.27mg	56%
Total Carbohydrates 64.62g	22%
Fiber 16.95g	68%
Sugar 23.17g	
Protein 9.26g	19%
MyPoints 6.48	

Recipe Tips

This recipe is perfect for any occasion. CONDIMENTS CAN DESTROY A DIET! Let's discuss condiments such as ketchup, mayonnaise, etc. The condiments that people use often add hundreds if not thousands of calories in a week's time. Read the calorie counts and decide if it's really worth it.

Zero Calorie Dressing

A simple and tasty dressing. As served at FitBodyRetreat.com.

4 tsp   Bragg Liquid Aminos   4 tsp   rice vinegar

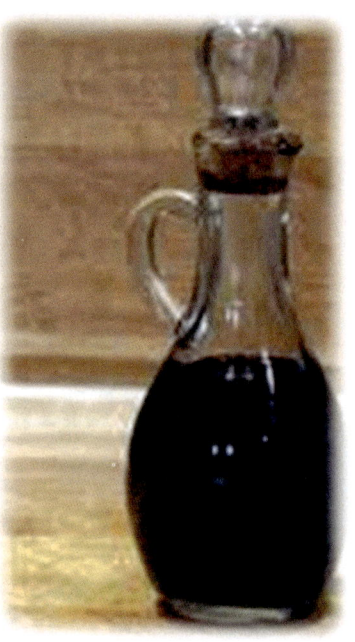

Procedure

1 Mix together and pour on salads.

Servings: 1

Preparation Time: 15 minutes
Cooking Time:
Total Time: 15 minutes

Nutrition Facts

Serving size: Entire recipe (1.4 ounces).

Amount Per Serving	
Calories	2.8
Calories From Fat (0%)	0
	% Daily Value
Total Fat 0g	0%
Sodium 641.43mg	27%
Potassium 142.8mg	4%
Total Carbohydrates 8.42g	3%
Protein 4g	8%
MyPoints 0.06	

Recipe Tips

This stuff is the best! I had an intern from Australia, who stayed at our center for 3 months, teach me this salad dressing. ZERO calories – well, almost zero. Thanks Jules! I use this every day. Caution -- way too many people will make a wonderful salad and then destroy it with 500 calories of processed blue cheese dressing. Use this stuff and your salad will get none of the extra poison or calories associated with the processed dressings that you find at the store.

Everything Thai

The Grand Lodge

I was fortunate to have trained in a Thai restaurant kitchen while in boxing in Thailand several years ago with my oldest son Dan. Here you will find a few of my favorite Thai recipes. In particular, the Thai salad and Green Lipstick Soup are our client's favorites.

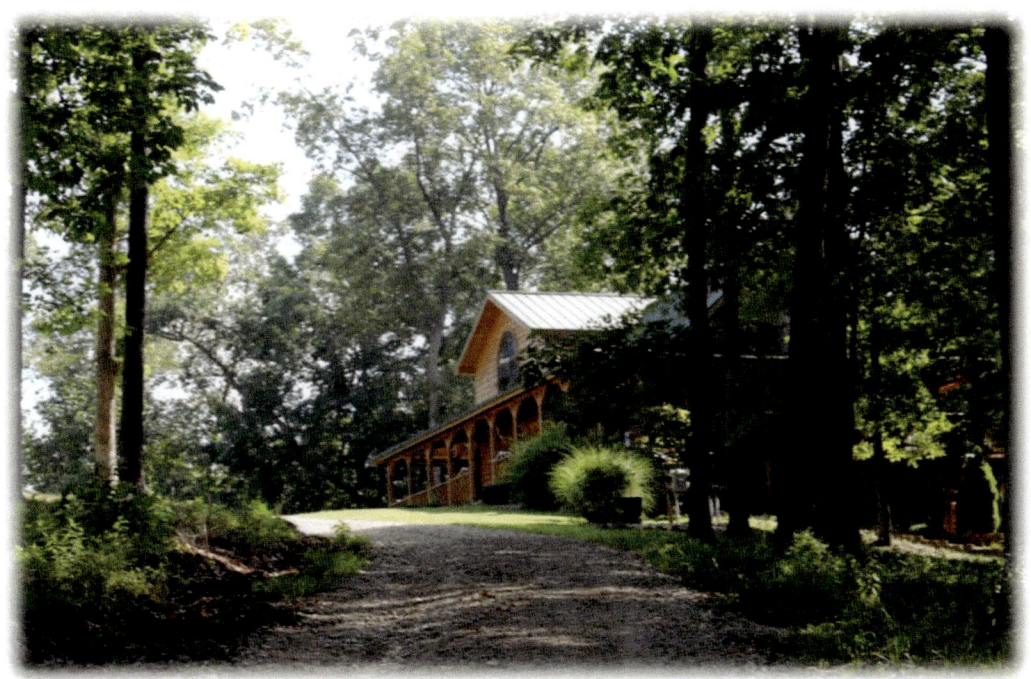

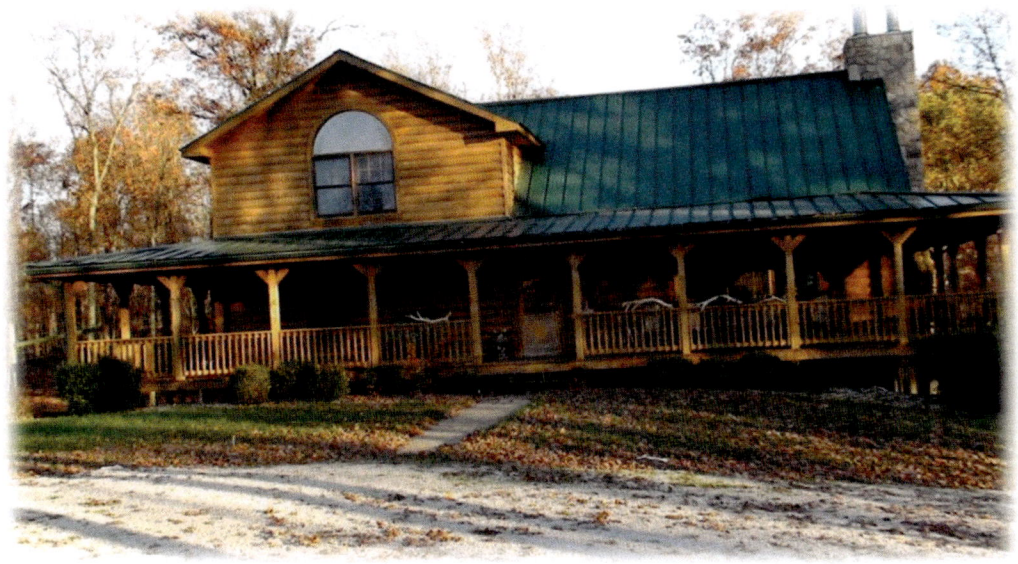

Chicken Satay

Delicious as an appetizer or main entry! As served at FitBodyRetreat.com.

2	handfuls	sliced chicken, cubed tofu, scallops, shrimp, pork, beef, etc. (about 2 cups)	1	tsp	oyster sauce
			1	tsp	agave
			4	tbsp	macadamia nut oil
2	tsp	garlic, chopped	1	ea	red pepper
2	tsp	yellow curry powder			
1	tsp	Bragg Liquid Aminos			

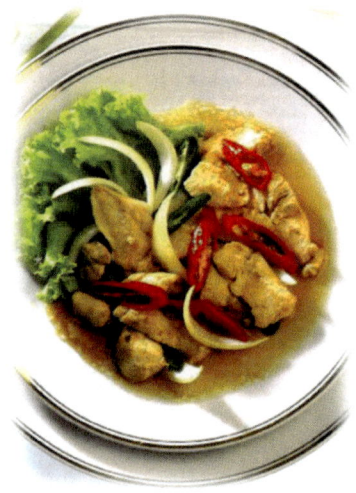

Procedure

1. Mix all ingredients together in a bowl.
2. Fry in a non-stick pan until done.

Servings: 2

Preparation Time: 10 minutes
Cooking Time: 10 minutes
Total Time: 20 minutes

Nutrition Facts

Serving size: 1/2 of a recipe (10.7 ounces).

Amount Per Serving	
Calories	518.5
Calories From Fat (66%)	343.07
	% Daily Value
Total Fat 37.8g	58%
Saturated Fat 2.6g	13%
Cholesterol 105mg	35%
Sodium 275.9mg	11%
Potassium 517.41mg	15%
Total Carbohydrates 6.79g	2%
Fiber 2.26g	9%
Sugar 3.13g	
Protein 36.7g	73%
MyPoints 13.07	

Recipe Tips

I make this dish a lot! It is so easy and so good! You really want to serve it up with a peanut sauce though. Be careful which sauce you buy. Some are high calorie. I use about ½ a teaspoon or 30 calories for my personal use. I learned this dish while kick boxing in Thailand with my oldest son Dan.

Spicy Fruity Thai Sensation

A delicious, fruity, sweet, sour, hot dish that was created here at the ranch using proven Thai cooking principles. As served at FitBodyRetreat.com.

2	tbsp	oyster sauce	1	ea	pear
1	tbsp	Bragg Liquid Aminos	1	ea	avocado
1	tbsp	hot sauce (Sriracha or rooster sauce)	1	ea	mango
4	tbsp	agave	1	ea	lemon, juiced

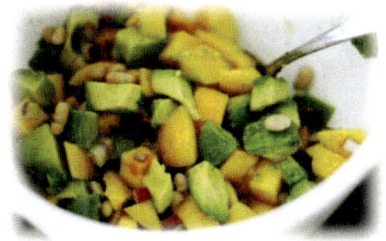

Procedure

1. Cut up fruit into small squares.
2. Combine all ingredients into a bowl or container with lid.
3. Squeeze the juice from 1 lemon onto it.
4. Shake or stir all together. (I prefer to shake)
5. Serve in a small cocktail dish.

Servings: 6

Preparation Time: 10 minutes
Cooking Time:
Total Time: 10 minutes

Nutrition Facts

Serving size: 1/6 of a recipe (11.1 ounces).

Amount Per Serving	
Calories	131.55
Calories From Fat (41%)	53.68
	% Daily Value
Total Fat 4.66g	7%
Saturated Fat 0.65g	3%
Cholesterol 0mg	0%
Sodium 327.14mg	14%
Potassium 256.22mg	7%
Total Carbohydrates 13.62g	5%
Fiber 3.49g	14%
Sugar 7.98g	
Protein 1.59g	3%
MyPoints 2.32	

Recipe Tips

See why wine is good for you? I created this delicious recipe after being over-served on some red wine one night with clients at the Oasis! You will love it. Sweet, sour, hot, and spicy!

Thai-Garlic Chicken

Simple and tasty! As served at FitBodyRetreat.com.

2	handfuls	chicken breast, thinly sliced (about 2 cups)	1 tsp	Bragg Liquid Aminos
2	tsp	garlic, chopped	1 tsp	agave
1	tsp	oyster sauce	1/8 tsp	white pepper
			2 tsp	macadamia nut oil

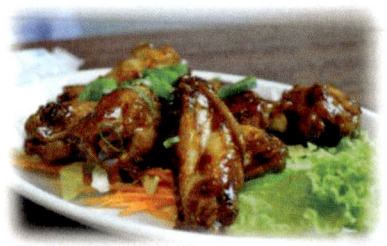

Procedure

1. Mix all ingredients together except for the oil.
2. Add oil to non-stick pan on medium heat.
3. Add all ingredients to pan and cook until done.

Servings: 1

Preparation Time: 10 minutes
Cooking Time: 10 minutes
Total Time: 20 minutes

Nutrition Facts

Serving size: Entire recipe (14.5 ounces).

Amount Per Serving	
Calories	435.48
Calories From Fat (37%)	160.63
	% Daily Value
Total Fat 16.72g	26%
Saturated Fat 1.62g	8%
Cholesterol 181.44mg	60%
Sodium 662.8mg	28%
Potassium 1074.86mg	31%
Total Carbohydrates 2.71g	<1%
Fiber 0.21g	<1%
Sugar 0.06g	
Protein 61.66g	123%
MyPoints 10.06	

Recipe Tips

I don't care whether it's wings, breasts or thighs, or whatever other part of the chicken you choose. This will be a favorite recipe! Pork works well with this recipe too.

Thai-Green Curry Soup

Hot! "Bring a sweat on Curry Soup that everyone who likes spicy foods will enjoy!" As served at FitBodyRetreat.com.

1 tbsp	extra virgin olive oil	1/2 can (15 oz)	chicken stock, lite, low sodium*
2 handfuls	chicken (or any meat - about 2 cups)*	2 ea	kaffir lime leaves
		3 tbsp	fish sauce, low sodium*
2 tbsp	green curry paste	2 tbsp	agave
2 handfuls	snow peas		
2 can (13.5 oz)	coconut milk, lite*		

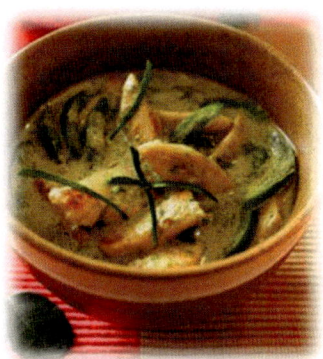

Procedure

1. Place oil, meat and curry paste in a non-stick pan.
2. Cook until meat is about 1/2 done.
3. Add the coconut milk and chicken stock.
4. Add snow peas and remaining ingredients.
5. Bring to a boil.
6. Simmer until the snow peas are done, about 3 min if you want them firm.

Servings: 4

Preparation Time: 10 minutes
Cooking Time: 10 minutes
Total Time: 20 minutes

Nutrition Facts

Serving size: 1/4 of a recipe (19.5 ounces).

Amount Per Serving	
Calories	281.45
Calories From Fat (64%)	181.32
	% Daily Value
Total Fat 16.9g	26%
Saturated Fat 0.87g	4%
Cholesterol 45.36mg	15%
Sodium 1042.69mg	43%
Potassium 262.27mg	7%
Total Carbohydrates 5.48g	2%
Fiber 0g	0%
Sugar 0.75g	
Protein 15.52g	31%
MyPoints 7.04	

Recipe Tips

I learned all the Thai dishes in this cookbook while boxing in Thailand. I make this particular dish more than the others. If you want it to cause a runny nose, just double the green curry. If you want fewer calories, use lite coconut milk. I often make it with salmon and scallops rather than chicken.

* You can use regular coconut milk and chicken stock instead of the lite version in this recipe. However, if you're trying to limit calories, use lite.
* If you want the soup thicker, use less chicken stock.
* You can substitute fish sauce with Bragg Liquid Aminos for a healthier alternative.
* My favorite meats in this soup are salmon cubes, scallops, or shrimp. Chicken is good too.

Thai-Herb Salad

Hot, spicy and yummy! Perfect salad that hits all the flavors. As served at FitBodyRetreat.com.

1	handful	cabbage, savoy (about 2 cup)
1/2	handful	carrots, sliced thin like matchsticks (about 1/2 cup)
1/2	handful	cucumber, peeled and sliced thin like matchsticks (about 1/2 cup)
1/2	ea	tomato, cubed
2	ea	Thai shallots (or any shallots)
1/2	handful	red chili peppers, sliced think like matchsticks (about 1/2 cup)*
1/2	handful	lemon grass, chopped (about 1/2 cup)
1	tbsp	extra virgin olive oil
1	tbsp	Bragg Liquid Aminos
1	tbsp	oyster sauce
1	tbsp	agave
2	tbsp	lemon juice

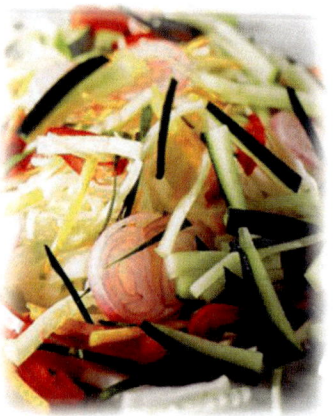

Procedure

1. Mix all together in a bowl.
2. Add lemon juice last.

Servings: 2

Preparation Time: 15 minutes
Cooking Time:
Total Time: 15 minutes

Nutrition Facts

Serving size: 1/2 of a recipe (14.7 ounces).

Amount Per Serving	
Calories	177.46
Calories From Fat (39%)	69.64
	% Daily Value
Total Fat 7.32g	11%
Saturated Fat 1.01g	5%
Cholesterol 0mg	0%
Sodium 548.28mg	23%
Potassium 675.01mg	19%
Total Carbohydrates 20.41g	7%
Fiber 4.27g	17%
Sugar 6.71g	
Protein 5.09g	10%
MyPoints 3.36	

Recipe Tips

I make this at my center every week. It's a spicy favorite. All who try it seem to like it.

* When I can't find a good hot chili pepper, I'll use Sriracha or rooster sauce

Thai-Spicy Easy Fish

Hot and spicy. Easy to make. As served at FitBodyRetreat.com.

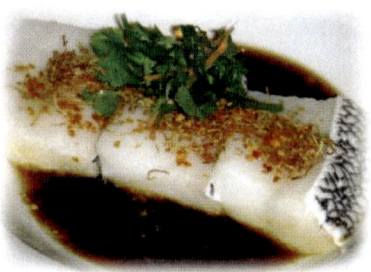

The Base
- 1 ea — cod fillet (or any white fish)
- 1 tsp — macadamia nut oil
- 1/2 tbsp — green curry
- 2 tsp — garlic, chopped
- 1 tsp — oyster sauce
- 1 tsp — Bragg Liquid Aminos
- 1 tsp — agave
- 1 tsp — white pepper

The Sauce
- 4 tsp — water
- 2 tsp — agave
- 2 tsp — fish sauce
- 2 tsp — oyster sauce
- 2 tsp — lemon juice
- 1 tsp — macadamia nut oil

Procedure
1. Place fish and oil in a non-stick pan with the green curry.
2. Add remaining ingredients to pan, except for sauce, and mix well.
3. Mix sauce ingredients in a separate bowl.
4. Place fish on 1/2 the sauce, and place remaining 1/2 of sauce on top of fish.

Servings: 1

Preparation Time: 10 minutes
Cooking Time: 10 minutes
Total Time: 20 minutes

Nutrition Facts

Serving size: Entire recipe (23.4 ounces).

Amount Per Serving	
Calories	365.48
Calories From Fat (32%)	118.49
	% Daily Value
Total Fat 11.03g	17%
Saturated Fat 0.33g	2%
Cholesterol 99.33mg	33%
Sodium 1997.47mg	83%
Potassium 1033.18mg	30%
Total Carbohydrates 8.1g	3%
Fiber 0.83g	3%
Sugar 0.75g	
Protein 43.63g	87%
MyPoints 8.06	

Recipe Tips

If you notice the ingredients, almost all Thai dishes contain the same stuff!

Detox Protocol

Home Detox Kit

6-Day Detox

If you choose to do a detox on your own, we can send you the supplies that you'll need to do it privately in your own home. This particular detox is quite aggressive though. It is best advised to do it at a center with supervision.

What's included in the kit

54 Chompers	3 Chompers 3x per day = 9 x 6 days = 54
36 Herbal Nutrition	2 Herb Nutrition 3x per day = 6 x 6 days = 36
12 Probiotics	2 per day x 6 days = 12
6 Multi-Vitamin Packets	1 packet daily x 6 days = 6
20 tbs Spirulina	3 tsp 3x per day = 9 tps x 6 days = 20 tbs
72 drops Stevia	4 drops stevia per spirulina drink x 3 = 12 x 6 days = 72 drops
24 tbs Psyllium	1 tbs 4x per day x 6 days = 24
24 tbs Bentonite Clay	1 tbs 4x per day x 6 days = 24
12 Smooth Move Tea	1 bag 2x per day x 6 = 12

Supplies you will need to buy

9 lemons	½ lemon juice per spirulina drink 3 x per day = 1-1/2 lemons daily x 6 days
organic coffee	1 pot of organic coffee per colonic bucket (most people do 1 colonic daily – some do 2)
1 lg grapefruit	
2 onions	
6 carrots	
4 potatoes	
2 cups parsley	unchopped
4 stalks of celery	
1 qt of water	
1 bottle of Bragg Liquid Aminos	

Broth Ingredients

1 onion

3 lg carrots

2 potatoes

1 cup parsley (unchopped)

2 stalks celery

½ qt water

1 tbs Bragg Liquid Aminos

Directions

Bring to a boil

Let simmer for 1.5-2 hours

Strain broth

Drink one bowl at 6:00pm (dispose of the vegetables)

This will make enough broth for 3 days. Make second batch on day 3 or 4.

Smooth Move Teas

Drink 1 cup of tea 2x per day

Steep tea for 10 minutes before drinking

Note: Drink as much lemon water daily as you wish (except on liver flush day)

Liver Flush Ingredients

½ cup olive oil

4 tbs epson salt

1 large grapefruit

Spirulina Drink

You will drink 3 of these drinks daily—see schedule

1 tsp. spirulina

½ juice from ½ lemon

4 drops stevia

Blend in a blender and drink

Liver Flush Recipe

Epson Salt Component

You will drink 2 of these drinks on day 5 in the evening and 2 on day 6 in the morning so a total of 4 epson salt drinks--- see schedule

  1 tbs. epson salt
  ¾ cup water

Combine ingredients and drink quickly

Olive Oil Component

  ½ cup olive oil
  Juice from 1 grape fruit

Combine ingredients, shake well and drink

Liver Flush Schedule

Day 5 - No liquids of any kind after 2:00pm (this includes no broth)

6pm   Drink the first epson drink

7pm   Drink the second epson drink

9pm   Drink the olive oil/grapefruit drink

7am   Drink the third epson drink

8am   Drink the fourth epson drink

9am   Drink water as usual

Psyllium Shake

You will drink 4 of these shakes daily- see schedule

  1 tbs psyllium
  1 tbs bentonite clay
  1 sprinkle cinnamon
  ¾ cup water

Combine ingredients, stir and drink quickly. Add 3 drops of vanilla stevia for flavor if you need it.

Colonics

This detox protocol requires a minimum of 1 colonic every other day. Plan on 4 colonics over the course of 6 days with the last colonic on day 6. If you wish to have a professional colon hydro-therapist help you with your colonics, schedule some appointments in advance. If you are not planning on doing colonics, then I recommend that you do not attempt to do this detox. Choose a different detox program. The colonics are a key element of this program.

What each of the herbs look like:

Chompers = brown capsules
Herbal Nutrition = green capsules
Probiotic = white pill
Multi-Vitamins = packet of vitamins

Daily Schedule

7am   spirulina drink

7am   (Chompers, Probiotics, Herbal Nutrition) Herbs

8am   psyllium shake

10am psyllium shake

11am spirulina

12pm (Chompers, Probiotics, Herbal Nutrition) Herbs/ Vitamin Packet

3pm   psyllium shake

5pm   psyllium shake

6pm   broth

7pm   spirulina

7pm   (Chompers, Probiotics, Herbal Nutrition) Herbs

Recipe Index

Recipe Index

A

A Bit of Green	187
Almond Nut Milk	54,190
Asparagus	118

B

Basil Grilled Chicken	68,94
Basil Pesto	152,191
Bean Salad	136,192
Bearnaise Sauce II	164
Beef Stew	69,95
Berries & Yogurt	34,174
Black Beans Basic	119
Breakfast Burritos	35
Breakfast Quinoa	36
Breakfast Tacos	37
Brown Rice	120
Buffalo Salsa Wrap	70
Burrito Protein Power House	71

C

Carrot, Apple & Green	22,55,193
Ceviche	72
Chicken & Red Pepper Wrap	73
Chicken Caesar Wrap	74
Chicken Satay	96,226
Chicken Tofu Pizza	75
Cinnamon Apple & Almond Ricotta	175
Cocoa Almond Drink	56,194
Coconut Rice & Mango	176
Coconut Sweet Potato or Yam	121
Cottage Cheese with Banana & Flax	38
Curry Split Pea Soup	137

D

Dave's Favorite Raw Dressing	165,195

E

Eggs Easy & Quinoa	39
Elk & Lentil Burritos	76
Elk Chili	77
Elk Garlic BBQ Burger	78
Elk Meat Loaf	97
Energy Soup	138,196

F

Fage 2% Yogurt, Granola & Fresh Fruit	40
Fish Cakes	79
Flaxseed Blueberry Pancakes	41
Forbidden Black Wild Rice	122
French Toast	42
Fresh Mango Yogurt	177
Fresh Tomato Parmesan Scramble	43

G

Garlic Teriyaki Edamame & Chicken	98
Ginger Cucumber Salad	139,197
Ginger Salmon Salad	140
Ginger Salmon with Wild Rice	99
Greatest Detox Vegetable Broth	23
Green Algae Drink	24,57,198
Green Beans	123
Green Smoothie & Berries	25,58,199
Green Veggie Juice #1	26,59,200
Green Veggie Juice #2	27,60,201
Grilled Wasabi Salmon	100
Growing Sprouts & Making Rejuvelac	28

H

Hard Boiled Eggs & Hummus	153
High Power Smoothie	61
High Protein Chips & Salsa	154
High Protein Oatmeal	44
High Protein Pancakes	45
Himalayan Red Rice	124

I

Iced Herbal Coffee	62

L

Lemon Herb Chicken	101
Lentil Soup	141
Lentils Basic	125
Lentils with Tomatoes	126
Lettuce Tofu Veggie Wraps	80
Lettuce Veggie Wraps	81,202
Liver Flush	29

M

Mediciettes, Steak Appetizer with Bearnaise Sauce	102
Mexican Flax Crackers	155,203

O

Oaties & Scramble / Pico-de-Gallo	46

P

Peanut Butter Chocolate Banana Oatmeal Post Workout Shake	186
Perfect Filet Mignon	103
Pico-de-Gallo	156,166,204
Pork Tenderloin	104
Prime Rib Tenderloin	105
Protein Bars	157
Protein Omelet	47
Psyllium & Bentonite Clay Drink	30

Q

Quinoa and Edamame Salad	142
Quinoa Basic	127
Quinoa Curry	128
Quinoa Curry & Chicken	106
Quinoa, Beans & Elk	82

R

- Raw-Alfredo Sauce 167,205
- Raw-Apple Sauce 178,206
- Raw-Berry Cheesecake 179,207
- Raw-Chocolate Avocado Mousse 180,208
- Raw-Fajita Alternative 83,209
- Raw-Garden Burgers 84,210
- Raw-Ice Cream Sundae 181,211
- Raw-Oatmeal Cookies 182,212
- Raw-Ranch Dressing 168,213
- Raw-Smokey Jalapeno Cheese Alternative.. 158,214
- Raw-Sour Cream 169,215
- Raw-Taco's Tasty Meat Alternative 159,216
- Raw-Zucchini Pasta 85,107,217
- Real Orange & Fresh 63,218
- Red Pepper Stuffed & Chicken Salad 86
- Red Skin Potatoes Roasted 129
- Rice Pasta - Gluten Free, Wheat Free 130

S

- Salmon & Cucumber Quinoa Salad 108,143
- Scrambled Eggs with Cottage Cheese 48
- Scrambled Eggs with Feta & Veggie 49
- Scrambled Eggs with Goat Cheese & Red Peppers 50
- Seared Ahi Tuna 109
- Seaweed Mineral Drink 31,64,219
- Shrimp & Rice Penne Pasta 110
- Snow Peas 131
- Spaghetti Sauce 170
- Spaghetti Squash with Chicken Breast 111
- Spicy Black Bean Soup 144
- Spicy Fruity Thai Sensation 183,220,227
- Spinach Salad 145
- Spinach, Cabbage & Tuna Salad 146
- Spinach, Pepper & Cheese Salad 147
- Spinach, Wilted with Mushrooms 132
- Steamed Broccoli 133
- Super Post Workout Shake 186

T

- Thai-Garlic Chicken 112,228
- Thai-Green Curry Soup 148,229
- Thai-Herb Salad 149,230
- Thai-Spicy Easy Fish 113,231
- Turkey & Fruit 114
- Turkey Sandwich 87
- Turkey Sandwich - Multigrain 88
- Turkey-Elk-Buffalo-Beef Burger Grilled 89
- Typical Replacement Shake 187

V

- Veggies & Hummus Dip 160,221

W

- Wasabi Salmon 115
- White Chili - Turkey 90

Z

- Zero Calorie Dressing 171,222

Made in the USA
Coppell, TX
31 October 2020